WILD RESCUES

A PARAMEDIC'S *EXTREME ADVENTURES* in

YOSEMITE, YELLOWSTONE, and GRAND TETON

KEVIN GRANGE

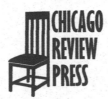

CHICAGO
REVIEW
PRESS

Published by Chicago Review Press
814 North Franklin Street
Chicago, Illinois 60610
ISBN 978-1-64160-200-6

Library of Congress Cataloging-in-Publication Data
Names: Grange, Kevin, author.
Title: Wild rescues : a paramedic's extreme adventures in Yosemite,
  Yellowstone, and Grand Teton / Kevin Grange.
Description: Chicago : Chicago Review Press, 2021. | Summary: "Wild
  Rescues is a fast-paced, firsthand glimpse into the exciting lives of
  paramedics who work with the National Park Service: a unique brand of
  park rangers who respond to medical and traumatic emergencies in some
  of the most isolated and rugged parts of America. In 2014, Kevin Grange
  left his job as a paramedic in Los Angeles to work in a response area
  with 2.2 million acres: Yellowstone National Park. Seeking a break from
  city life and urban EMS, he wanted to experience pure nature, fulfill
  his dream of working for the National Park Service, and take a crash-
  course in wilderness medicine. Between calls, Grange reflects upon the
  democratic ideal of the National Park mission, the beauty of the land,
  and the many threats facing it. With visitation rising, budgets shrinking,
  and people loving our parks to death, he realized that-along with the
  health of his patients-he was also fighting for the life of "America's Best
  Idea."— Provided by publisher.
Identifiers: LCCN 2020050398 (print) | LCCN 2020050399 (ebook) |
  ISBN 9781641602006 (trade paperback) | ISBN 9781641602013 (pdf) |
  ISBN 9781641602020 (mobi) | ISBN 9781641602037 (epub)
Subjects: LCSH: Grange, Kevin. | Park rangers--United States--Biography.
  | Emergency medicine--United States--Biography. | Emergency medical
  services--United States--Biography. | Rescues--United States--Biography.
Classification: LCC SB481.6.G73 A3 2021 (print) | LCC SB481.6.G73
  (ebook) | DDC 363.6/8092 [B]--dc23
LC record available at https://lccn.loc.gov/2020050398
LC ebook record available at https://lccn.loc.gov/2020050399

Cover and interior design: Preston Pisellini
Cover photo: AP Images
Back cover photo: Kevin Grange

Printed in the United States of America

5 4 3 2 1

For the park rangers, past, present, and those in the future,
who keep "America's Best Idea" alive

CONTENTS

AUTHOR'S NOTE

IN THIS MEMOIR, I have changed the identifying details of patients and, in some cases, the exact location of the emergencies described to protect individuals' privacy. However, the nature of the emergency calls and the treatments I provided have not been altered. In addition, out of respect for the privacy of National Park Service personnel—and since many work in law enforcement and are involved in active investigations—I have changed their names and identifying details and, in some cases, have created composites of their personalities. I did not change the names of the medical directors with whom I have worked since they are well-known public figures, and I thought it important to honor their great work and contributions to emergency medicine within our national parks.

To date, I've worked on a seasonal basis at Yellowstone, Yosemite, and Grand Teton National Parks. While pinballing back and forth is a great adventure for the seasonal employee, it can be difficult to follow for a reader. To account for this, I have condensed the time I spent at these parks into separate sections in the book and organized the emergencies according to call type and sometimes generalized dates, times, and order of events. I have also included some 9-1-1 calls that I responded to with Jackson Hole Fire/EMS in the national forests surrounding Grand Teton, since they share the same wild, remote nature.

Lastly, this book represents my own personal views and does not represent the views of the US Department of the Interior or National Park Service. The events and conversations depicted here are based on my own recollection, and I've worked hard to ensure the details are accurate. I take full responsibility for any inaccuracies.

My hope is for *Wild Rescues* to provide readers with a sense of the rigorous job that remote and rural first responders endure and to increase awareness and appreciation for our national parks and the dedicated people who work there. If this book kindles your interest in the National Park Service, I encourage you to explore working in a national park as either a volunteer or paid employee. Above all, my hope is for *Wild Rescues* to inspire you to enjoy our national parks with your family and friends. Get outside and never stop exploring our vast, beautiful planet!

—KG

PROLOGUE

RETURN OF SPONTANEOUS CIRCULATION

If a trail is to be blazed, send a ranger. If an animal is floundering in the snow, send a ranger. If a bear is in a hotel, send a ranger. If a fire threatens a forest, send a ranger. And, if someone needs to be saved, send a ranger.
—STEPHEN T. MATHER, first director of the National Park Service

THE FIRST TIME I helped bring back someone from a cardiac arrest in a national park occurred at 4:39 pm on Saturday, April 4, 2015.

An hour earlier, Erwin Barret, a fifty-six-year-old cattle farmer from Wisconsin, was having a heavenly day. It was the first time he'd visited Yosemite, and as he drove into the valley with his wife, Rebecca, and their twenty-eight-year-old son Jake, he couldn't get over the magnificent waterfalls and the granite monoliths of El Capitan and Half Dome rising above the fog-blanketed forests. After lunch, Erwin and his family decided to hike around the rocks of Lower Yosemite Falls. Hoping for a better view of

America's tallest waterfall, which tumbles 320 feet from the high crags in two successive steps, Erwin scrambled to the top of a large boulder. But as he stood up, something about the dizzying scale of the granite cliffs and the sound of water crashing in all directions threw him off balance. Jake attempted to catch his father, but instead they both fell ten feet into the shallow water and boulders below.

When the call came in, I was scarfing down a turkey wrap in the EMS office at the Yosemite Medical Clinic. I'd missed lunch when I went out on a search-and-rescue (SAR) mission up the Mist Trail earlier that day for an elderly woman who'd fainted.

"Ambulance 3," the dispatcher called over the radio, "please respond to the rocks beneath Lower Yosemite Falls for a report of two people who fell off a boulder."

Standing, I squeezed the last bite of my sandwich into my mouth and hurried to the ambulance.

Luke Cohen, a park law-enforcement ranger, arrived on the scene first. If you were ever ill or injured in a remote place like Yosemite, Mount Rainier, or Zion, Luke was the person you wanted responding. He perfectly embodied an "all-hazards" responder and was everything I aspired to be. Along with being a park ranger and paramedic, he was also highly trained in structure fire, wildland fire, search and rescue, and hazardous material emergencies; and he was certified in tactical EMS, high-angle rope, and swift-water rescue. Like some kind of special-ops soldier, he was able to operate in all environments—earth, air, and water—and was just as comfortable dangling out of a helicopter performing a short-haul rescue on the side of El Capitan as he was plucking a drowning victim from the Merced River's swift current. Best of all, Luke was a calm and consummate professional, no matter what the emergency. But when he gave his scene size-up over the radio that afternoon, his voice sounded panicked.

"I have two patients," he said, struggling to catch his breath, "one green tag, one red."

Color-coding patients as green, yellow, red, or black tag was a way to quickly triage, or sort, patients in a multiple-casualty incident. A "green tag" meant the patient could walk and had minor wounds. A "yellow" patient was more severely injured, and a "red tag" meant the victim had critical, life-threatening injuries. A "black tag" meant call the coroner.

"Ambulance 3 copies update," I replied. "Arriving on-scene."

Noah, my partner on the ambulance that afternoon, and I parked at the trailhead, grabbed our spinal immobilization equipment and basic life support bag—which had oxygen, splinting equipment, bandages, and curved, plastic devices known as "airway adjuncts" so patients didn't choke on their own tongues—and raced up through the boulders and shallow water.

As we approached, I spotted the telltale signs of an emergency—a body lying supine, surrounded by worried bystanders who appeared helpless. Fortunately for the patient though, Luke was also on-scene.

"This is Erwin," Luke announced as we arrived, gesturing to an overweight man in jeans and a red Wisconsin Badgers football shirt. "About fifteen minutes ago, he fell into the water from approximately ten feet, from that boulder just behind us. Family states he had a loss of consciousness lasting approximately one minute. They, along with a few bystanders, helped drag him from the shallow water, and now he's alert but says he can't move or feel his lower extremities. I also noticed he's growing increasingly lethargic."

Luke had started an IV in Erwin's right arm, covered him with a silver emergency blanket to prevent hypothermia, and placed a cervical collar around his neck. But Erwin didn't look good. He was pale and shivering, and his body was wedged between two boulders. His eyes were closed, and he kept whispering, "Please help me."

"Hang in there, Dad," said Jake, "We're doing everything we can."

Miraculously, Jake had suffered only minor bruises and abrasions during the fall. He stood next to his mother.

As other search-and-rescue team members arrived, adorned in bright yellow shirts, helmets, and black radio harnesses, we quickly moved Erwin to a rigid backboard and carried him through the boulder field. We suspected Erwin had a brain bleed and a high thoracic spinal injury, either of which could kill him at any moment.

"Coming through!" I yelled at a throng of tourists snapping pictures on the footbridge. "Emergency!"

By then, we'd placed Erwin onto the gurney and were wheeling him down the paved path toward the ambulance.

"Go with Dad in the ambulance," Jake instructed his mother. "I'll drive over and meet you at the landing zone."

"OK," she replied, hurrying to the front passenger's seat.

In the back of the rig, we cranked the heat and removed Erwin's wet clothes. Next, we obtained a set of vital signs and performed a detailed physical assessment. Erwin had a three-inch, hatchet-like laceration on the back of his head and an open gash on his right forearm . . . but we weren't blinded by bright, bloody things. His altered mental status and lower-limb paralysis were what concerned us the most.

"Stay with us Erwin," Noah said, pinching his shoulder. "Can you open your eyes for us?"

"Please . . . help . . . me," Erwin managed, his voice growing fainter.

"Start driving!" I yelled to the ranger at the wheel.

The ranger upfront gunned it for Ahwahnee Meadow, five minutes away, where we'd meet a medevac helicopter. Luke had requested one as soon as he'd arrived on-scene and realized Erwin was critical.

As we started driving, dodging potholes on the bumpy road and launching off frost heaves, I leaned my head toward the front to give Rebecca an update on her husband. I told her about the interventions we were performing to help Erwin. "We're warming him to prevent hypothermia. We've started an IV to give him warm saline, checked his vital signs, EKG, and blood sugar. We've also dressed his wounds, and he's doing a lot better."

Of course, no sooner did I say that than Erwin decided to die on us.

"Stop the ambulance!" Noah yelled. "He coded!"

The driver slammed on the brakes as I began CPR. Erwin's belly bounced in a wave-like fashion with each compression, and I heard a few ribs snap like zip ties. This was quite normal when you performed high quality CPR on older patients, but it was always hard to hear.

When Erwin lost his pulse that afternoon, Noah, Luke, and I quickly leapt into action. We focused all of our energy on a series of tasks that, when performed perfectly and paired with a few milligrams of good luck and epinephrine, just might bring about a return of spontaneous circulation.

As I performed chest compressions, Noah slapped defibrillation pads on Erwin's chest, and Luke inserted an airway adjunct, so Erwin didn't swallow his tongue, then delivered breaths with a bag valve mask.

A moment later, Erwin moved slightly, and we detected a heartbeat.

"I've got a pulse!" Noah yelled up to the driver. "Let's go!"

The ranger gunned it toward Ahwahnee Meadow, but, seconds later, Erwin's eyes glazed over again.

"Stop the ambulance!"

We started CPR a second time and, within moments, Erwin's pulse returned again.

"Drive!"

The driver hit the gas.

"Stop!"

Rebecca was beside herself in the front seat. *Stop! Go! Stop! Go! Alive! Dead! Alive! Dead!* Such was the back-and-forth roller-coaster ride of running a cardiac arrest.

When I started to tire, we switched positions, and Luke began compressing on Erwin's chest while Noah managed the airway. I scanned Erwin's arm for a second IV site but couldn't locate one easily. I wasn't going to spend any time fishing around, so instead I drilled an intraosseous needle directly into the marrow of Erwin's shinbone, allowing us to infuse fluids and medication directly into his venous system.

A moment later, Erwin blinked his eyes open again.

"Drive!" Noah yelled again.

Erwin retained his pulse for the remainder of the short drive, but we feared he had a high-thoracic spinal cord injury, which was causing these intermittent respiratory—and cardiac—arrests.

We arrived at Ahwahnee Meadow to find a landing zone set up and secured by a team of firefighters wearing yellow bunker gear. While we waited for the helicopter to arrive, we obtained another set of vital signs, obtained a 12-lead EKG to take a detailed look at Erwin's heart rhythm, and gave him the medication Zofran for nausea.

"Head injury patients are airway obstructions waiting to happen, because they vomit," Luke reminded me.

The air ambulance arrived a few minutes later, appearing over Half Dome in the bright sunlight. Seeing the helicopter, ambulance, fire engine, and multiple patrol vehicles, all the tourists watching assumed absolute hell was breaking loose. But we knew it was just another day in one of America's national parks where anything could happen—and often did.

"Good luck, Erwin," I said, as we loaded him onto the bird and transferred care to the flight crew. "They'll take good care of you."

• • • • • • •

After the helicopter lifted off, bound for a Level 1 trauma center in Fresno—two and a half hours in the ambulance, but only thirty minutes by air—and the law enforcement units and fire engine cleared, a quiet calm returned to Yosemite Valley. We debriefed after the call—what went well, what we could improve—and then returned to the clinic to replace the equipment on our ambulance. Once everything was restocked, we radioed dispatch that we were back in service.

The call was officially over, but it did not end there. At least not for me.

Like a coach watching the game tape, I spent the rest of the day—and most of the night—reviewing every moment of the incident and asking myself: *Did I miss anything? Could I have done anything different? Or worked faster? Was there anything I should've checked but didn't? Did I provide compassionate care?* I knew I'd never run the perfect call, but that didn't mean I wouldn't spend my whole career aspiring to.

As the night wore on, my thoughts drifted to my experiences as a paramedic and park ranger with the National Park Service. During my time working for the NPS, I had responded to an unresponsive scuba diver in Yellowstone's Firehole River, a heart attack victim in the spurting shadow of Old Faithful, various rock climbing falls, drug overdoses, stroke patients, and multiday search-and-rescue missions.

Around 1:00 am, my worried thoughts started to abate. The images swirling in my mind grew fuzzy, like a camera out of focus, and I began to drift off to sleep. And it was about that time that law enforcement rangers spotted a man down in the meadow across from El Capitan.

A dispatch voice sounded in the dark—"All units stand by for a page for Ambulance 3"—and then shrill alarm tones blared from my pager as it vibrated and rattled across my nightstand like a chattering teeth windup toy.

I threw on my uniform and ran to the rig.

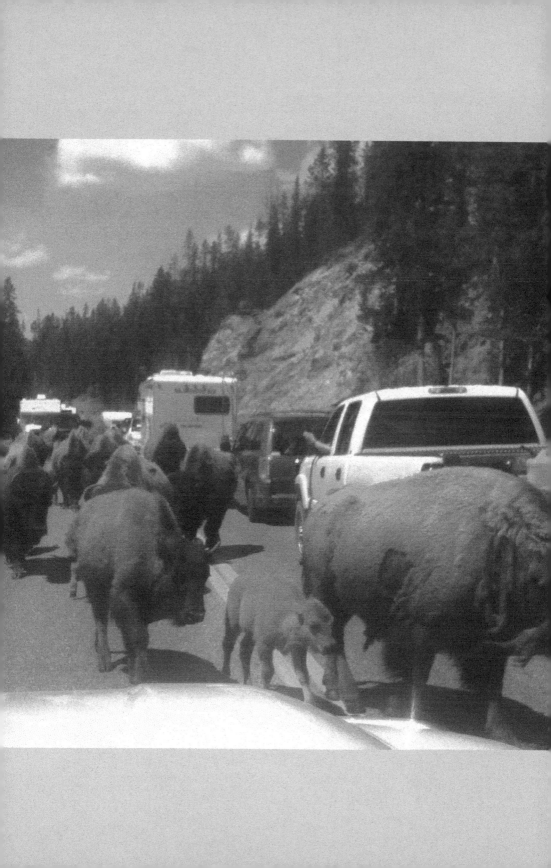

PART I

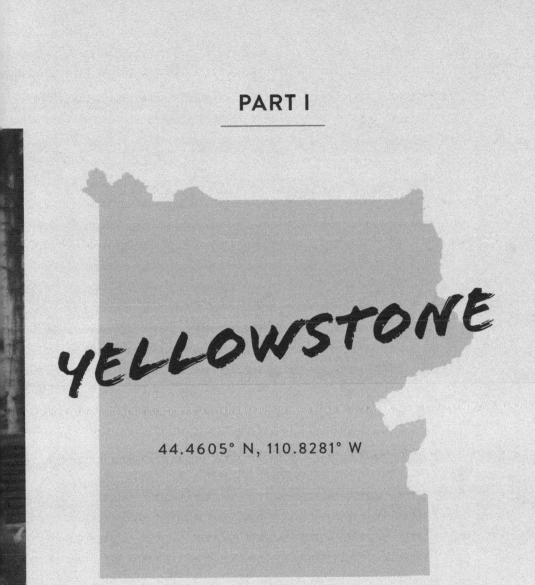

YELLOWSTONE

44.4605° N, 110.8281° W

I went to the woods because I wished to live deliberately, to front only the essential facts of life, and see if I could not learn what it had to teach, and not, when I came to die, discover that I had not lived.

—Henry David Thoreau, *Walden*

1

THE DEFINITION OF INSANITY

MY WILD ADVENTURE with the National Park Service began long before that traumatic cardiac arrest call in California's Yosemite National Park. The first national park I worked at was Yellowstone, which occupies parts of Wyoming, Idaho, and Montana. I arrived there from Los Angeles during a snowstorm in early May 2014. (Yes, they have snowstorms up there even in May.) I hadn't even stepped out of my car before the first 9-1-1 call came in. As I parked in front of the Old Faithful Ranger Station, the apparatus bay opened, and the ambulance slowly emerged, its emergency lights turning the white snow globe that surrounded me red and blue.

Spotting my California plates in the near-empty parking lot, the driver rolled down the window and gestured. "You must be the new paramedic," she yelled above the squall. "We have a call!"

Was this an invitation? Or a warning about the busy summer that awaited me? Either way, I quickly parked and sprinted to the ambulance, hopping in the back.

"I'm Kevin," I hollered as we drove.

"Emily," the driver said loudly, glancing in the rearview mirror. "And this is Cody!"

Emily Wilde worked as Old Faithful's fire officer. She was in her early thirties, with brown hair, freckles, and a friendly smile. Cody Riley, a grizzled guy in his late forties, sat in the front seat next to her.

The rest of our introductions would have to wait. There was a sixty-eight-year-old woman with dizziness and a racing heart at the visitor center who needed our help.

"I'll take lead," Cody said, pulling on a pair of blue exam gloves. "Emily will get a set of vital signs, and I want you to place the patient on the cardiac monitor so we can look at her EKG."

"Copy," I replied, catching my reflected smile in the side window. I was about to run my first call in a national park and couldn't have been happier. Months earlier, I had been working on an ambulance in Compton, California, and my life was at a dead end.

After working for years in the restaurant and real estate industries, I'd signed up for an EMT class at age thirty-five, hoping to help people in a more direct and meaningful way. An EMT certification was the bare minimum for someone operating on an ambulance, and the class consisted of 120 hours of instruction in providing basic life support on emergency calls that ranged from broken bones and cuts to diabetic emergencies, heart attacks, strokes, and cardiac arrest.

From the moment I walked into my first EMT class, I knew I'd found my calling. I loved everything about prehospital medicine—the challenge and unpredictability, the unique blending of critical thinking with practical skills, the team-based approach, and of course, running all the crazy calls and helping people. Hoping to deepen my knowledge base—and become certified to operate at the highest level—I attended UCLA's Paramedic Education Program. Paramedic school was 1,500 hours of didactic instruction, written exams, high-stress skills stations, and a grueling field internship with a local fire department or EMS agency that many students described as "the best time in my life that I'd never want to repeat again." Along with basic life support, as paramedics we were trained to provide advanced life support by placing IVs, inserting breathing tubes, administering dozens of medications, and using a cardiac monitor to speed up, slow down, or restart a patient's dying heart.

I'd assumed things would get easier after attending paramedic school—the hardest physical and mental thing I'd ever done—but as soon as I stepped off the graduation podium, I'd taken my place at the back of a long, serpentine hiring line composed of thousands of men and women who, like me, sought firefighter paramedic jobs in Los Angeles. I hadn't prepared at all for the hiring process to be so competitive—or to take such a long time. There were over ten thousand applicants when I applied to the Los Angeles Fire Department for an initial recruit class of seventy firefighters, and the hiring cycle took months.

With no other options, I accepted a paramedic job with a private ambulance company in Compton. Our headquarters was located on Kona Drive, just off Mahalo Place. The street names brought to mind Maui's sunny beaches and bottomless mai tais, but I quickly learned that in reality, it was merely a drab area of industrial buildings. And when you took a right on Central Avenue and crossed over the 91 Freeway, the Compton I'd long heard about on rap albums emerged: single family homes with barred windows, liquor stores, and gang graffiti along palm-tree-lined streets like Crenshaw, Slauson, and Rosecrans Avenue—as famous (and notorious) as the hip-hop artists who sang about them.

"Just don't get out of the ambulance alone," my partner warned.

At the private ambulance company, we occasionally provided mutual aid and 9-1-1 response for the Compton Fire Department—when gang life got "hot" and the number of patients exceeded their supply of ambulances—but mainly we handled simple transports, like taking patients from nursing facilities to dialysis clinics, convalescent homes to community hospitals, or halfway houses to psychiatric wards.

While I enjoyed helping people and interacting with my patients, the hours were long, the pay was low, and the scene was never safe. My partner and I were often sent alone into LA's worst neighborhoods, where our dark blue uniforms and silver badges made us look a lot like cops. Our back muscles strained and tore from struggling to lift morbidly obese patients with a team of two, and we were routinely exposed to methicillin-resistant Staphylococcus aureus (MRSA), clostridium difficile (C-diff), feces, and scabies, microscopic bugs that lay eggs in the upper layer of skin. Nurses would send us into patient rooms, claiming we didn't need any isolation precautions, but then arrive at the bedsides after us wearing protective gowns, gloves, face masks, safety glasses, and surgical caps.

We picked up schizophrenic patients on involuntary psychiatric holds—threatening to kill themselves and others—along with tattooed prisoners from Twin Towers Jail downtown, the largest correctional facility in the world. Once we arrived at one of the rundown community hospitals where we transported our patients, we often had to wait for hours in the hallway to get a bed. "Holding up the wall" with a patient for hours at a time was common; my record was seven hours, on one particularly busy Monday.

In between transports, we waited for the next assignment by "posting" our ambulance in empty lots and city parks frequented by prostitutes and drug dealers. In addition to the tedium, since I wasn't running 9-1-1 calls anymore, I wasn't using the full extent of the training that I'd received at UCLA, and I feared I was losing the quick and efficient patient assessment skills I'd worked so hard to achieve.

Along with having a crappy ambulance gig, I was also broke. The fire department jobs for which I was applying required me to make—and pay for—repeated trips across the country for written exams, work capacity tests, interviews, polygraphs, and drug tests. And as if that all wasn't enough, my girlfriend, Chantal, broke up with me. My job difficulties reminded her too much of her deadbeat ex-husband, she said, and she'd lost respect for me.

Chantal had slammed the door in my face, refusing to talk, and then assumed a cross-legged seat on her yoga mat and started chanting for the peace and happiness of all sentient beings.

"Please, Chantal," I'd pleaded. "Just let me back in."

"Ommmmmmmm . . . Ommmmmmmm . . . Ommmmmmmmm . . ."

"We can work this out!" I said.

"Ommmmmmmm . . . Ommmmmmmm . . . Ommmmmmmmm . . ."

In short, I was at a low point in my existence, both personally and professionally. My life felt like the standstill traffic on the 405 Freeway.

But everything changed one November morning with the sound of snow chains.

I was camping with my parents in California's Yosemite National Park. An unexpected snowstorm had blanketed the Sierras, so we were relaxing in our RV, sipping coffee, and playing cards while admiring the Narnia-like snowy splendor that surrounded us. I'd just laid down three aces in a game of gin rummy when I heard the hum of a diesel engine and the rattle of snow chains hanging off a rear axle. I looked out the window and spotted an ambulance, painted white with a forest-green stripe, belonging to the National Park Service. The park ranger, a handsome guy in his late twenties, smiled and waved. He was a shepherd, checking in on his flock after the freak snowstorm. I waved back and he continued on.

Until that moment, it had never dawned on me that there were paramedics serving in our national parks, responding to medical and traumatic emergencies in some of the most remote and wild parts of the United States. However, given the isolation, dangerous terrain, inclement weather, and abundance of things that bite, claw, and sting, it certainly made sense.

"Now there's a job you should get," my dad said.

I couldn't believe I hadn't thought of it myself.

Although I was living in Southern California at the time, I'd grown up on forty-six acres in New Hampshire. Family camping trips were a staple of my childhood, and I'd once dreamed of being a ranger after encountering one in Moose Brook State Park when he'd stopped by our tent to politely ask us to quiet our laughter since it was after 10:00 pm.

Questions immediately fluttered around in my mind. *What kind of emergencies did a national park paramedic run? How was it working in a wild, remote area with the closest hospital hours away? Running an emergency call with limited personnel?*

I suspected there was a whole new side of the paramedic profession I hadn't yet witnessed.

"I'd love to work here," I exclaimed.

I needed a change. Working for the private ambulance service and applying to fire departments in Los Angeles and elsewhere felt like an endless treadmill of disappointment, and working for the National Park Service seemed like an ideal reset button.

"It's the perfect plan," I told my parents. "I'll do a season with the Park Service while I'm waiting to get hired by a department in LA."

In the weeks that followed, I researched emergency medical services with the NPS. With over four hundred units in the National Park System, spread out across our country like natural, cultural, and historical diamonds, I discovered EMS was handled quite differently at each. The smaller park units (such as historic sites, national seashores, monuments, and preserves) typically delegated fire and EMS response to outside agencies serving the gateway towns that bordered them. But the bigger parks—like the Grand Canyon, Lake Mead, Mount Rainier, or the Great Smoky Mountains—had robust fire, EMS, and search-and-rescue programs and operated their own ambulances, staffed by rangers who were EMTs and paramedics, or park medics, a variation of the two.

The certification levels for EMS providers were an ever-evolving and often confusing subject. In brief, emergency medical technicians could provide basic life support (BLS) interventions like controlling bleeding, splinting, operating an automatic external defibrillator, providing oxygen, and assisting with medications like aspirin for a heart attack, glucose for a diabetic patient with low blood sugar, or epinephrine for a bad allergic reaction. Along with BLS care, advanced life support providers such as NPS park medics and paramedics could insert a breathing tube down a patient's windpipe, start IVs, use a cardiac monitor to treat abnormal heart rhythms, and administer dozens of medications.

Most of the paramedic jobs with the NPS were summer seasonal positions starting in May and lasting into October. If candidates performed well, they were eligible for rehire status and often hired to work at other parks. The NPS was like the Mob in that way: once you were in, you were in.

As I read about the positions, I could barely contain my excitement. The paramedics (or "healthcare technicians," in government speak) would "spend minimal time indoors or behind a desk" and would respond to the usual array of medical and traumatic emergencies—stroke, seizures, heart attacks, broken bones, allergic reactions, and diabetic emergencies—in an "out of hospital/field setting." Due to the extreme environment and "frontier medicine" aspect of the job, they would also be asked to treat patients who were potentially suffering from heat exhaustion, heat stroke, burns, frostbite, hypothermia, lightning strikes, or insect bites, along with a distinct category ominously described as "injuries caused by wildlife." The job notice warned that the climate could be "as extreme as the activities that are available" noting that the incumbent might be expected to fly in a helicopter, or stay overnight with a patient in a backcountry setting, or perform collateral duties such as search and rescue, fight wildland or structural fires, provide visitor assistance and education, and handle resource management.

If hired, I would wear the classic uniform of a park ranger—green duty pants and a gray collared shirt adorned with the National Park Service arrowhead on the right sleeve, along with the brass badge and the iconic, broad-brimmed hat. In addition to saving lives, my duty would be to uphold the Organic Act of 1916, which pledged to leave the scenery, wildlife, and natural and historic objects "unimpaired for future generations." As a federal employee, I would take an oath of office and solemnly swear "to support and defend the constitution of the United States against all enemies, foreign and domestic" and to accept the position with "true faith, allegiance, and without any mental reservation."

As someone who grew up loving the outdoors, I was excited about these responsibilities and felt it would be a great honor to uphold them.

When spring approached, I eagerly applied for jobs at Lake Mead, Grand Teton, Grand Canyon, Yosemite, and Yellowstone. Despite my enthusiasm, I found applying to these positions as frustrating as all the others I'd been pursuing: my resume wasn't formatted to the strict National Park Service standard, my answers to the job questionnaire were insufficient, I got referred for a job but then not asked to interview, or I got an interview but wasn't selected for the position.

Months passed, then a year, and my situation in Southern California grew more dire. When the private ambulance shut down their paramedic division, I was forced to work as an EMT to pay my bills. By then, I felt my career hadn't just stalled but was moving in reverse. Now, I could no longer start IVs, analyze patients' EKGs, or treat their pain with a narcotic like morphine or fentanyl. I could only provide the bare minimum of basic life support. I had serious concerns about my future in EMS.

I was on the verge of giving up my dream when my phone rang one afternoon in March 2014 with the offer of a position in Yellowstone's iconic Old Faithful district. Along with the Yosemite Valley and the South Rim of the Grand Canyon, Old Faithful was one of the busiest districts for EMS and law enforcement contacts in all of the National Park Service.

"We figured you could handle the call volume and craziness since you're from Los Angeles," Rachel Johnson, Old Faithful's district ranger, explained over the phone. "You probably won't see gang shootings, but we do have bison gorings and bear maulings."

I suddenly realized I was about to be a character out of BBC's *Planet Earth*.

"I'll take it!" I exclaimed immediately. Six weeks later, I said goodbye to family and friends and found myself north on I-15, bound for the Cowboy State of Wyoming.

LAND OF LARGE CARNIVORES

I GUNNED IT TO SALT LAKE CITY, spent the night, then continued north into Idaho, passing potato farms and tiny towns. As I drove, I listened to country singer Eric Church and mentally reviewed Yellowstone's treatment protocols. Since I'd be working in an austere and remote environment with the possibility of prolonged field care and long transport times to the hospital, my scope of practice would be much wider than any intervention I was ever asked—or allowed—to perform in Los Angeles at the time. For example, I could execute a risky procedure known as a needle cricothyrotomy, which involves passing an over-the-needle catheter into the cricothyroid membrane—the notch just below the Adam's Apple (thyroid cartilage)—if I couldn't ventilate a patient or place a breathing tube due to massive trauma or swelling of the airway. If I were unable to insert an IV, I could also drill into a bone to obtain vascular access, and my medication box would be filled with drugs rarely seen in a city: the antibiotic ancef, to give critical trauma victims; ketamine, for pain or to sedate combative psychiatric patients; and diltiazem, to slow down dangerously fast and irregular heartbeats.

There were also treatment protocols for every imaginable environmental emergency—heat stroke, hypothermia, frostbite, drowning, altitude sickness—and even one for "Accidental Exposures to Wildlife Immobilization Agents," in case one of the biologists accidentally shot themselves with the highly-potent tranquilizers they carried to subdue bears or bison. In addition, there were the protocols about what not to do. In Los Angeles at the time, nearly every trauma patient who took even a mild fall was placed in a cervical collar and rigid backboard. However, since it wasn't uncommon to transport patients for over two hours in Yellowstone, we rarely used rigid backboards, which could cause severe discomfort and pressure ulcers. Instead, we'd decide on whether to place our patients in full spinal precautions or to employ the use of a "vacuum mattress" which formed to the patient's body and was a lot more comfortable than a rigid backboard.

As I drove, I felt like all the disparate elements of my life were finally coming together. Yet as I passed through Rexburg, Idaho, my enthusiasm dropped like the service bars on my cell phone. I'd done my research prior to my deployment and knew that Madison Memorial in Rexburg was the closest medical facility to Old Faithful. A glance down at Google Maps revealed I still had 112 miles to go until I arrived at my summer post. The closest hospital with a trauma center that could also treat patients having heart attacks or strokes? Eastern Idaho Regional Medical Center in Idaho Falls, over two and a half hours away from the legendary geyser. In California terms, it was the equivalent of picking up a critical trauma patient in Los Angeles and "racing" them to San Diego. Sure, there was always the option of flying a patient out in a medevac helicopter or fixed-wing airplane, but that too was contingent on the moody mountain weather.

As I continued north of Highway 20, I found myself looking at Rexburg in my rearview mirror, not unlike how a sailor venturing forth into stormy seas might gaze wistfully back at shore.

It was an overcast and drizzly afternoon in early May, and as Highway 20 entered the dense woods of Targhee National Forest, in a winding ascent toward West Yellowstone, the rain changed to sleet and then, suddenly, I found myself in a snowstorm. I hadn't expected this but soon learned it wasn't uncommon to experience all four seasons—sun, rain, sleet, and snow—in a single day at Yellowstone. Like the locals said, "If you don't like the weather, just wait five minutes."

As I continued, semis barreled past in the opposite direction, as if fleeing, and sprayed my window with blinding slush. I couldn't see any mountains yet, but I felt their looming presence in all directions. I was in the wild country now. I could sense it in the impenetrable strands of pine trees and A-frame construction of cabins; in the bear-proof garbage bins and roadkill; and, as I stopped to get gas, in the way the local boys sized me up. I hadn't expected snow and was woefully underdressed in a T-shirt, shorts, and flip flops. The local guys were hulking, elk-fed men with beards, dressed in camouflage and Carhartt work pants. They drove raised pickups with gun racks and thick-treaded tires, and they gazed at me with a mixture of amusement and pity. While I'd grown up in New Hampshire, hiking and camping with my family and had always loved the outdoors, I couldn't help but feel I'd grown a bit soft since moving to California and living by the beach. Now I was a thousand miles from the ocean, a fish out of water, a fawn approaching the wolf den.

Eventually, I entered the park at West Yellowstone—a tiny gateway town of souvenir shops, old-time photo booths, and backcountry outfitters. It was really snowing by then, and as I drove slowly down the west entrance road, I had the sense of venturing forth onto another planet. Every now and then, through snow squalls, I'd catch a fleeting glimpse of dark, rolling mountains, bubbling hot springs, and sharp-horned beasts.

My first and only previous experience with wilderness medicine had occurred four years earlier on the twenty-four-day Snowman Trek in the Himalayan kingdom of Bhutan, a tiny country wedged between Tibet and India. I'd fallen in love with Bhutan, a country that governs by a unique policy of "gross domestic happiness," when I first visited in 2004. I returned three years later to hike the Snowman Trek for the first time and, soon after, was asked to guide the trek on two additional occasions. In 2010 I was leading the trip, when one of my hiking clients almost died from a lethal combination of dehydration and altitude sickness at thirteen thousand feet. The patient—a wife and mother of three from Australia—couldn't descend to lower elevation by hiking or riding a horse down because she was nearly unconscious. We called for a medevac helicopter on a satellite phone, but the closest "bird" was in India, over a hundred miles away and couldn't fly due to bad weather. With night fast approaching, my Bhutanese porters and I made a makeshift litter out of a backpack and logs and attempted to carry the woman to a lower elevation, but a snowstorm forced us back to camp. By then, the woman was nearly dead. Every now and then, she'd mumble her husband's name and then drift off again.

"We're going to have a body on our hands if something doesn't change," another of our hikers said.

When we returned to camp, we slid the woman into a portable altitude chamber, a pressurized bag that is meant to simulate the physiological effects of descending six thousand feet and helps improve oxygen exchange in the lungs.

At 3:00 AM, the woman was still on the verge of death, so I stepped outside the wooden hut to say a prayer. "Please, God, don't let her die," I pleaded, in the shadow of Mount Chomolhari, the 24,035-foot peak that was Bhutan's most sacred peak. "If you spare her life and help get this mother and wife home to her family," I prayed, "I promise I'll pay it back somehow."

By the next morning, through a combination of the portable altitude chamber, medications, and oral rehydration solution, the woman had miraculously improved. We were able to evacuate her the following day and, a few months later, I made good on my promise to God. I never wanted to be unprepared again. I wanted to learn to save lives at the highest level. I decided I would follow the one spiritual practice that held all life as sacred and believed that no one was beyond saving; that didn't care about a person's religion, skin color, sexual orientation, or income.

I enrolled in paramedic school.

· · · · · · ·

During that trek in Bhutan, I'd been lucky that both an internal medicine physician from Stanford and an ER nurse from England had been on the trip with me, but was I up to the challenge on my own? As I pulled up to the Old Faithful Ranger Station that first night—a dark wood oasis in the blowing snow—there was no time to ponder the question as I spotted the ambulance pulling out of the apparatus bay.

I'd be working with a team of law enforcement rangers, paramedics, and volunteers at Old Faithful, but since it was still early May, many hadn't arrived yet.

Emily, Cody, and I wheeled the gurney through the visitor center and found the patient in a small room next to the information desk. Virginia, a frail woman from New Mexico, was struggling to breathe and had anxious eyes. As Cody inquired about her medical history, Emily and I quickly obtained a set of vital signs and an EKG. We discovered the woman's pulse racing at nearly three times the normal speed, a potentially lethal dysrhythmia called supraventricular tachycardia (SVT). Her heart was beating so fast, it didn't have enough time to fill back up with blood.

"That's why you're feeling short of breath and dizzy," Cody explained to her.

He handed her an empty 10cc syringe and instructed her to bring it to her mouth and exhale through it until the plunger moved. The hope was that this vagal maneuver would stimulate her vagus nerve, a cranial nerve that connects the brain to the body and could convert her heart rhythm back to normal naturally. Virginia drew in a deep breath and exhaled as Cody encouraged her: "Keep going . . . keep going . . . exhale . . . exhale!"

Virginia's face flushed with effort, and the plunger slowly moved. Moments later, her heart rate magically dropped back to normal on the cardiac monitor.

"Wow! I feel better," Virginia said, dabbing a handkerchief to her forehead to wipe away the perspiration.

Despite her improved condition, Cody still recommended she go to the hospital, which, by then, I knew was basically two states away: starting from Old Faithful in Wyoming, the ambulance would exit the park in West Yellowstone, Montana, before arriving a couple hours later in Rexburg, Idaho. Virginia agreed, and we assisted her onto the gurney and into the ambulance.

"Want me to ride in back?" I asked Cody, knowing he would still have to start an IV, hang a bag of normal saline, repeat the 12-lead EKG and monitor her vital signs continuously.

"I got this," Cody replied confidently, "Go settle into your apartment. We have a busy week ahead."

"What if she goes back into SVT?" I asked.

Cody said if that happened, he'd try another vagal maneuver or push a medication called adenosine. I knew a side effect of adenosine could be a pulseless rhythm called asystole—a flatline!—but there was something so tested and confident in Cody's tone that all my fears disappeared.

"Copy," I replied.

Cody wasn't the clean-shaven, polished brand of medic I'd worked with in Los Angeles; the kind who arrived on-scene with a large crew and an armada of parade-ready apparatus. He was grizzled, rugged, and autonomous, like a cross between an ER physician and Indiana Jones.

Even though I'd only just met him, I knew that I wanted to be just like Cody. I resolved to learn as much as I could from him and the other rangers I'd be working alongside at Old Faithful that summer, although I knew I would have to battle with a high-altitude, steep learning curve before I became nearly as skilled at remote wilderness medicine.

"Be safe out there," I said, closing the back door and waving to Emily.

The tires made a crunching sound on the snow as the ambulance slowly pulled out and disappeared down the road, leaving me alone in the fading light. Outside the Old Faithful Ranger Station, the American flag whipped in the wind, and in the distance, a coyote called out, its mournful howl echoing in the white void.

THE WORLD'S FIRST
NATIONAL PARK

ON MARCH 1, 1872, President Ulysses S. Grant signed the Yellowstone National Park Protection Act into law, creating the world's first national park "for the benefit and enjoyment of the people." With 3,472 square miles spread across Wyoming, Montana, and Idaho, Yellowstone is larger than Rhode Island and Delaware combined and welcomes over 3.5 million tourists annually, who come to witness the park's geothermal wonders, mountains, rivers, lakes, and abundant wildlife. Often called "America's Serengeti," the park is home to three hundred species of birds, sixteen species of fish, five species of amphibians, six species of reptiles, and the largest collection of mammals in the lower forty-eight states. Wolves, black bears, grizzly bears, fox, bison, moose, bighorn sheep, bobcats, and mountain lions—they're all here, along with pronghorn, elk, and mule deer that travel hundreds of miles over ancient overland routes in a grand migration that rivals Africa's wildebeests and the caribou of the Arctic.

Each May, a similar migration occurs as thousands of summer seasonal employees and volunteers flock to national parks across the United States. These summer workers support full-time National Park Service personnel in dozens of staff positions, from leading campfire talks and education programs to maintaining trails, conducting research, handling maintenance, staffing entrance stations and visitor centers, and working as law enforcement rangers, paramedics, and firefighters in the Visitor and Resource Protection Division.

Since it was early May, many of the seasonal employees hadn't arrived yet, and after I watched the ambulance depart from Old Faithful that first snowy night, I drove to my apartment in the government area—a cluster of townhomes, concessionaire employee dorms, and RV spots, hidden off the Grand Loop Highway that traverses the park in a big figure eight. I'd been assigned Unit B in an eight-plex, a row of single-story, one-bedroom apartments reserved for the Old Faithful ranger cadre.

The front door to my unit was unlocked, so I stomped snow from my flip flops and entered to find a modest living room and kitchen area, adorned with a small table and couch. Dropping my suitcase, I followed a short hallway past the bathroom and into the bedroom, where I discovered an empty gun safe in the closet and spare bullets underneath the bed. Had a law enforcement ranger resided there before me? Or had the previous tenant just known that being armed was a good idea in the land of large carnivores?

Despite being bone-tired, I hardly slept that night. Maybe it was the high altitude or the dry air—or the shoving match that went on all night between the wind and my apartment walls. Or maybe it was the stark realization that it was a long way back to the hospital, and the only thing standing in the middle of the thin red line between life and death here was me.

At dawn, I rose bleary-eyed, threw on my warmer clothes, and followed a snowy trail toward the visitor center. The storm had blown through, leaving clear skies and cold temperatures. From the government area, the trail bisected the Grand Loop Highway and passed the Old Faithful Ranger Station before crossing a large parking lot and arriving at the visitor center and Old Faithful Inn. Despite their close proximity, the visitor center and Old Faithful Inn were about as different as two buildings could be. Completed in 2010 at a cost exceeding $21 million, the visitor center had a state-of-the-art energy- and water-efficient design, built with recycled and eco-friendly materials. The center also boasted a 232-seat auditorium, a gift shop, and floor-to-ceiling pentagonal windows, through which guests could gaze at the world's most famous geyser.

By contrast, Old Faithful Inn had been built more than a century earlier, in 1904. It was the first of the great park lodges constructed in the West and was often referred to as a "wooden Sistine Chapel." The Inn resembled a seven-story-tall treehouse and featured a large stone fireplace, timber columns, hickory furniture, an antique clock, and polished pine railings.

On September 7, 1988, the Inn was nearly lost to fire. A lethal combination of lightning strikes, drought, and dry winds created the largest wildfire in Yellowstone's history, burning over 790,000 acres and leaving an apocalyptic image of downed, dead trees still seen today. As the conflagration was pushing toward the historic structure, Bob Barbee, Yellowstone's superintendent at the time, had closed the park, and firefighters hunkered down as the flaming front approached. With an Alamo-like determination, they'd switched the fire sprinklers into "deluge mode," draped fire hoses over the Inn, and took defensive positions. Overhead, helicopters and airplanes had conducted water drops to douse the blaze. Thanks to those brave and dedicated firefighters, no lives were lost, and Old Faithful Inn was saved.

As I kicked a trail between the Old Faithful Inn and the visitor center that frigid morning, I sensed something waiting for me on the other side and picked up my pace.

Moments later, I emerged into the winter wonderland of the Upper Geyser Basin, home to 60 percent of the world's geysers. Amidst rolling hills of glacial gravel and runoff channels, geysers hissed and spouted, mud pots bubbled like my grandma's beef stew, and steam shot up through cracks in the earth called "fumaroles." I'd never experienced such a dynamic landscape of fire and ice. The geysers smelled of sulfur and had mystical names like Castle, Grand, Daisy, Grotto, and Riverside. Suddenly, the queen herself, Old Faithful, woke up, bubbling for a hot minute before shooting water over a hundred feet in the air.

There were strange, magical forces at work beneath this ancient landscape, and I stood in awe. Some similarly subterranean impulse within me, felt but not entirely understood, had brought me to Yellowstone, and I would honor that. And then, as if to confirm that thought, the wind shifted, and I was sprayed with a warm baptismal mist from a roaring geyser named Beehive. All my worries disappeared. I thought, *Life's great when you're standing in geyser spray.*

· · · · · · ·

I spent the rest of the morning catching up with Cody. He was first in a long line of park rangers I'd meet who was an all-hazards responder and a total badass. This was Cody's third summer working as a seasonal paramedic in Yellowstone, and along with being a firefighter paramedic, he'd also worked as a ski patroller, as a wildland firefighter, as a search-and-rescue team member, and as a teacher for the National Outdoor Leadership School (NOLS). And he had extensive travel experience in the Himalayas.

Cody told me the craziest call he'd run was a grizzly attack, where the patient got scalped. "The bear was still on scene, so we had to wheel the patient out, who miraculously survived, with armed escort of two police officers, pulling security at the front and rear of the gurney, in case the grizzly charged again."

"Wow," I replied. "And I thought working as a paramedic in Compton was dangerous."

Cody said he'd also learned the hard way to never slice open a down jacket to expose a trauma patient. "The ambulance was filled with goose feathers!"

Around 3:00 pm, a white Ford F150 pickup with Texas plates roared up. It was another seasonal paramedic, Sam Simpson.

"Howdy, y'all," he said with a warm Lone Star drawl.

Sam Simpson was a good ol' Texan in his mid-fifties. When he wasn't spending summers in Yellowstone, Sam served as chief of the fire department in a small Texas town and owned a rafting company with his wife that ran trips on the Rio Grande through Big Bend National Park. Like Cody, Sam taught wilderness medicine for NOLS and also taught EMT classes for the US Border Patrol.

While Cody was an expert in winter emergency medicine, Sam was highly proficient in heat-related illnesses and injuries—no surprise, given that he lived in the desert. He'd been on numerous search-and-rescue missions, treating patients suffering from heat stroke or scorpion stings and snake bites, and since his town bordered Mexico, he'd delivered more than a few babies in the crooked shadows of prickly pear cacti. At the time, it was not uncommon for pregnant Mexican mothers to wait until they were in active labor to cross the border, having heard that a baby born on US soil received immediate citizenship. They certainly made Sam's job a bit more stressful.

Cody and Sam were as different as two medics who held the same certification could be. They both loved being outside, but Sam was outdoorsy in a country music kind of way—blue jeans, white T-shirt, a big brass belt buckle, and cowboy boots—while Cody was more of a Patagonia-puffy-jacket kind of outdoorsy. Still, I sensed they were the perfect pair to introduce me to wilderness medicine.

I said hello and introduced myself. Sam shook my hand and said, "Damn son, we're gonna have to fatten you up. You're as skinny as one of Yellowstone's lodgepole pines!"

"Lodgepole. Sounds like a perfect nickname to me," Cody added with a smile.

I laughed. I'd worked in EMS long enough to know that receiving a nickname and getting ribbed was a high compliment. It's when your coworkers stopped making fun of you that you had to worry.

Once we all finished getting settled in, we met on Sam's porch to sip whiskey and grill some steaks. By then, the temperatures had warmed, and the snow from the previous morning had melted.

After dinner, Sam handed out some Cuban cigars. With each of us holding a glass of whiskey in one hand and a stogie in the other, Sam made a toast.

"Gentlemen," he began, "Here's to a summer working in the most beautiful, magical places on earth."

Cheers!

ONBOARDING

WE MET BEFORE DAYBREAK the following morning and piled into the government vehicle we'd been issued for the week. It was a Chevrolet HHR, a retro, high-roofed station wagon. As we drove in the predawn gloom, dodging bison along the way, we decided "HHR" stood for "half a hot rod." We were heading toward the northwest district of the park, Mammoth Hot Springs. There, we'd stay in the red-roofed historic buildings of Fort Yellowstone, which had been built to house soldiers summoned in 1886 to discourage poaching, vandalism, and squatters within the park. In the shadow of travertine terraces stacked like limestone Legos, we'd spend the next several days at the annual EMS refresher. The refresher would be five days of attending lectures, performing skills stations, and running emergency scenarios in order to get credentialed, so that we could function as EMS providers within the park.

More than twenty EMTs, park medics, rangers, and paramedics from each of Yellowstone's eight districts attended the training, and each day followed a typical format: running through high-stress skills stations and emergency scenarios and learning about EMS operations in the park. After class we'd go for a group jog—dodging wandering elk and bison along the way—and then drive to grab dinner in the gateway town of Gardiner, Montana, passing under the famous Roosevelt Arch. There, in between bites of pizza and bison burgers, I'd hear from the longtime employees about the kinds of calls I could expect working in Yellowstone.

Some of the stories were especially horrifying: a three-year-old who accidentally shot herself while playing with her dad's handgun at Grant Campground; a California man who dove into a hot spring to rescue his dog, only to inhale boiling water and crawl out with his skin sloughing off and his eyes fried like egg whites; a concessions employee who was bench-pressing alone in the gym and let go of his weight bar when it was directly over his Adam's apple; an eight-year-old girl who lost her footing on a trail above the Grand Canyon of Yellowstone and fell five-hundred feet off a cliff; a forty-eight-year-old man who sustained a lethal massive head, neck, and chest injury after being gored by a bison; and a guy from Michigan who, in 2011, decided to hike alone on the Mary Mountain Trail. Unbeknownst to the solo hiker, he'd wandered into a "grizzly hole"—the term Wyoming residents bestowed on an area infested with the sharp-toothed bruins—where two bison carcasses wafted up their decaying scent like a Glade plug-in. His mauled body was found a few days later in an area with fifteen bear beds, shady spots where the bruins liked to spend the hottest part of the day. "There were significant lacerations to the left side of his head, including a laceration at the left corner of his mouth and a severe laceration to his left ear," the Board of Review report later concluded. "His body had been partially consumed and exhibited bite and claw marks consistent with attack by a bear." Along with these gruesome tales, there were also stories of drownings, car wrecks, and motorcycle accidents.

"But there's one behemoth lethal to both man and animal," Sam joked. "1-800-RV-4-RENT." There were more accidents involving RVs than any other vehicle in the park, although, fortunately, most were minor collisions in crowded parking lots.

Cody told me about Old Faithful's carcass dump and warned me never to go there if I ever found the coordinates of its top-secret location.

"It's the spookiest place in the park," Cody said, explaining that it was where law enforcement rangers—called LE rangers—and the maintenance crew dumped the dead elk, bison, and deer that had been killed by harsh winters, disease, or errant drivers. "The grizzlies hear the truck in the distance, and they come running."

"You never see the bears," Sam added, "but you can feel their eyes on you."

Cody said a visit to the carcass dump was so dangerous that maintenance crews only deployed there in teams: one getaway driver ready behind the wheel, one guy to discard the carcass, and a third standing ready with a gun in case a bruin charged.

Another ranger from Yellowstone's Lake District spoke of a cardiac arrest call he'd run where he had to cross the Firehole River in a small raft with all his equipment to reach his patient on the opposite shore. "And then, as we started working the patient up, this angry bison starts walking over!"

"Gives a new meaning to the term 'scene safety'!" quipped Cody.

At the end of dinner each night, I always had the same thought: *the myriad of Yellowstone's wonders is matched only by the many ways the park can kill you.*

Every hour of the EMS refresher was intense, and the stress level rose with each successive day. The credentialing process culminated that Friday, when each of us had to be a team leader during a simulated cardiac arrest call, then pass a written test, along with a rigorous oral board exam with Hugh Bensky, the EMS director, and Yellowstone's medical director, Dr. Luanne Freer.

"Have a seat there," Hugh said to me when it was my turn, gesturing to a chair across the table where he sat with Dr. Freer.

"Thank you, sir." I said, sitting.

I was exhausted after a long week of training and nervous as hell. Sam and Cody had informed me that more than a few medics had failed this part of the credentialing process and had been asked to pack their bags.

I was also extremely intimidated by the interviewers. Hugh Bensky had worked as an LE ranger and paramedic for over twenty-five years and was a legend within the NPS. Prior to Yellowstone, he'd worked at Denali National Park in Alaska, Ozarks National Scenic Riverway in Missouri, and Indiana Dunes National Lakeshore, near where he'd grown up in Indiana. Hugh had a warm, down-home Hoosier demeanor; he was so friendly that it was said criminals actually apologized to him for the inconvenience their arrests caused him. But he could also be as stern as a West Point drill instructor when it came to uniforms and appearances. No matter the late hour or 9-1-1 call, Hugh always wore his official park ranger uniform and never removed his flat hat. According to lore, he'd even worn his flat hat while performing an intubation—a difficult skill that required the provider to lay down on their stomach, inches from the patient's face, in order to insert a breathing tube into the patient's windpipe.

As for Dr. Freer, she was one of the world's foremost experts on high-altitude and wilderness medicine, having served as a past president for the Wilderness Medical Society. Along with being an

ER physician and medical director, her other "office" was perched at 17,500 feet above sea level on the world's highest peak, where she founded and ran Everest ER. In Yellowstone, she oversaw the three urgent care medical clinics in the Mammoth, Lake, and Old Faithful districts. Dr. Freer had been profiled by *Outside* magazine and Oprah Winfrey, and now she was interviewing me to work under her license as a paramedic at Yellowstone.

Hugh started by stating that the purpose of the oral boards was to test my ability to think on my feet and under pressure. "We want to hear how your approach a situation and assess and treat your patient. We also want to test your knowledge of our protocols, policies, and medications."

"Copy," I replied with a quivering voice.

Dr. Freer began by giving me a scenario where I'd been called to respond to the Fairy Falls Trail behind Grand Prismatic—a sprawling rainbow-colored hot spring for a fifty-five year old man severely short of breath. "You have ten minutes."

As we'd done in paramedic school, I began by telling Hugh and Dr. Freer that I'd first don safety glasses and exam gloves and ensure my scene was safe. "Next, I'm going to ensure his airway is patent; look, listen, and feel for breathing; and check his circulation by feeling his pulse and skin temperature."

Hugh informed me that we knew my patient's airway was clear because he was talking, but that he seemed to be struggling with his breathing, had a rapid respiratory rate, and that I could hear fluid rattling around in his lungs.

"I'll immediately apply oxygen via a non-rebreather mask," I replied, "and then obtain a set of vital signs and a 12-lead EKG to look for signs of a heart attack."

Dr. Freer told me the cardiac monitor didn't indicate a heart attack, but that my patient had an elevated blood pressure, a rapid heart rate, and that he was "80 percent oxygen on room air."

Hugh explained the man hadn't been taking his medications, especially his water pill, "because he's on a bus tour and doesn't want to have to go pee."

"You'll get that a lot here," added Dr. Freer.

Suddenly, all my nerves disappeared, and I found myself in the zone, that rare—and entirely welcome!—state of supreme focus in an EMS scenario.

"This man is suffering from left-sided heart failure," I said confidently before explaining that the left ventricle of his heart has lost the ability to contract normally, so blood is not circulating adequately through the body, and fluid is backing up into his lungs. "Therefore, we need to decrease the workload of his heart, dilate his vessels, and improve his oxygenation."

"How?" asked Dr. Freer, scribbling down notes.

I told them I'd use nitroglycerine to open up his vessels, apply a CPAP mask to force oxygen past the fluid into his capillaries, start an IV, and give him Lasix—if available—to lessen his fluid retention, then start transporting him.

"What's your destination?"

"The clinic at Old Faithful," I replied. "And if he deteriorates, there's a helipad out back where we can fly him out."

"Anything else?"

"That's it," I replied.

Dr. Freer and Hugh wrote more notes and tallied up my score.

"Decent," Hugh began. "But you have a lot to improve on."

That wasn't the enthusiastic feedback I'd been expecting.

Hugh reminded me that I needed to give a scene size-up over the radio after I had completed my primary assessment of checking the patient's airway, breathing, and circulation and determined his chief complaint. "This isn't like Los Angeles, where you always arrive with a cavalry. It might just be you or you and one other person. But all of the Old Faithful rangers are listening on the radio, so you need to let them know what you have and what you need."

Hugh also wondered how I planned on moving the patient to the ambulance.

"The gurney?"

"Not on that trail," he replied.

"Walking him?"

Hugh looked at me sternly. "A patient with heart failure and difficulty breathing?"

I admitted to them that I didn't know.

"A wheeled litter would be a good choice," Hugh said

I'd never even heard of the device, but evidently, I'd have to learn about it. Fast.

Dr. Freer said transporting the patient to the clinic at Old Faithful wasn't the right move either. "You never want to drive deeper into the park."

"But the Old Faithful Ranger Station has a helipad," I countered.

"What if the weather changes, and the helo can't land?" posed Hugh. "It happens frequently."

Dr. Freer said I should always be moving patients in the direction of definitive care. "In this case, that means driving toward the park entrance. You can use pullouts along the way to land a helicopter if needed or request a fixed-wing airplane to meet you at the airport in West Yellowstone."

"Yes, ma'am," I said. I'd gone from feeling like a "para-god," sure they would anoint me the greatest gift to medicine since Hippocrates, to being uncertain if I would even pass.

Hugh asked why I chose to perform all of my interventions—like starting an IV and performing a 12-lead—on-scene.

"I thought it would be easier than in a moving ambulance."

Hugh shook his head and said transport times in Yellowstone could be anywhere from forty-five minutes to nearly three hours. "Basic life support on-scene. Advanced life support and everything else en route."

Dovetailing off that, Dr. Freer asked me how much oxygen was in the main tank of the ambulance.

"I'm not sure."

"A CPAP device requires high-flow oxygen, and your patient could potentially be on the mask for hours," she warned. "Don't be one of those paramedics who runs out of oxygen on the way to the hospital. It's happened here, and it wasn't good."

By then, I was certain I'd failed. There was so much more than simply medicine to working in a remote setting.

Hugh looked at Dr. Freer, who nodded and then turned to me.

"You've got a lot to learn," she began, "but we think you have a good knowledge base and, if you continue to work hard, will be successful here."

"Welcome to Yellowstone," Hugh said, standing and shaking my hand. "Good luck!"

• • • • • • •

In order to be officially signed on and be able to act autonomously in the back of the ambulance, I still had to run a few calls and pass my field training with Sam and Cody, but as we returned to Old Faithful that Friday, I was relieved to feel like everything was coming together. The snow was melting, more seasonal staff and volunteers had arrived while we were away, and the once-sleepy government area now felt active and alive.

To celebrate, I threw my bear spray and park radio in my trail pack and took off for a run, passing the Old Faithful Inn and then following the paved path north. I ran past Castle, Daisy, and

Riverside Geysers, but once I reached Morning Glory hot spring, I stopped on the wooden viewing platform and watched steam rise from its scalding, tropical blue waters.

And that's when I saw it—the tawny brown fur, the shoulder hump, and the rounded "dish-like" face. A grizzly bear was crossing the Firehole River a hundred yards upstream.

A few tourists, standing beside me, snapped pictures. Freaking out and fumbling, I dove into my pack for my bear repellent and radio.

"Dispatch," I said, keying my radio. "We've got an emergency at Morning Glory. There's a grizzly!"

The dispatcher copied my radio traffic. "How far away is the bear?"

"About a hundred yards!"

"Is it approaching people?"

"No, ma'am."

"Are people approaching the bear?"

"Negative."

"Is anyone hurt?"

"No."

I heard what sounded like a sigh on the radio, and I could literally see the dispatcher rolling her eyes. "So you called to tell us there is a grizzly bear in Yellowstone National Park?"

I felt more than stupid. Even the tourists, city slickers from Boston, looked at me like I was crazy.

"Um yeah. I guess so."

"Are you in danger?"

I said no.

"Do you need additional resources?"

"Negative," I replied. "Sorry for wasting your time."

As I turned off my radio, the bear disappeared into the woods.

Cody, Sam, Emily, and the others were all waiting to poke fun at me when I returned to the government area. My radio transmission had been broadcast over the entire Old Faithful District. I felt like such an idiot.

That night, we held a big campfire and potluck at the communal fire pit. Everyone was there—LE rangers, interpretation rangers, trail crew, maintenance workers, wildland firefighters with thick bushy beards, and nurses in light blue scrubs from the Old Faithful Clinic.

"Welcome to adult summer camp," Cody joked.

"See this, Lodgepole?" Sam said, gesturing as he served me up a cheeseburger. "Old Faithful is a campfire community."

"What?" I replied, distracted as I hit "refresh" on my cell for the hundredth time. The cell phone service at Old Faithful was terrible. Since arriving, I'd come to realize I had a social media addiction. I'd almost had an existential crisis when I discovered I didn't get good reception. I used to live a life of "I post, therefore I am," Descartes be damned.

Sam gave me a look and repeated himself.

"A campfire community," I replied, ashamedly pocketing my phone. "Definitely." I resolved to stop focusing on my phone and be more present during my time at Yellowstone.

Sam said I could expect potlucks like this one nightly during the summer. "Just bring your pager in case a 9-1-1 call pops off," he explained. "And no drinking if you plan on responding on the ambulance."

As the evening wore on, I gorged on hot dogs, salads, and seven-layer dip and made the rounds, meeting people. I found them just about the most interesting, diverse, and friendly bunch of people I'd ever met. Backcountry Bill worked in the permit office at Old Faithful, handing out campsites, and looked like an icon from the Old West. His silver hair flowed to his shoulders from under his cowboy hat, and he sported a goatee and mustache reminiscent of Captain Jack Crawford, the "poet scout" and storyteller of the late nineteenth century. Fittingly, when his summer season at Yellowstone ended, Backcountry Bill spent winters at Bent's Old Fort National Historic Site in Colorado, where he played the role of a fur trapper trading with the Cheyenne and Arapahoe tribes in living history reenactments.

Will and Sarah were retirees from Alabama and devout Baptists who, despite being married for half a century, still doted on one another like newlyweds. They were participating in the Volunteers-In-Parks program. In exchange for volunteering thirty hours of their time at the Old Faithful Ranger Station each week, VIPs like Will and Sarah received a free RV spot in the government area.

Will was a retired police officer, and he offered his services as an ambulance driver any time I needed. "Day or night," he said kindly. "You know where to find me."

Another ranger, Zach Lang, had majored in ornithology—the scientific study of birds—before he became an LE ranger and park medic. He and Emily, the fire officer, lived together with their two dogs in a townhome adjacent to the eight-plex. A husband-and-wife pair of interpretation rangers, who worked at the visitor center and gave campfire talks, resided above them.

Anne Chen, the physician's assistant, and Jessica Schultz, the lead nurse, were both members of the clinic staff, who worked closely with us. We paramedics would transport those patients with urgent-care-type complaints to them, and in turn, they'd request our services to take patients who required a higher level of care to the hospital via the ambulance.

Sam and Cody told me there was a long history of Old Faithful rangers dating members of the clinic staff, and a few had even gotten hitched. However, Anne and Jessica were both already married. Their husbands planned to work remotely all summer—well, assuming the Wi-Fi ever worked.

Still reeling from a broken heart, I hadn't come to Old Faithful looking for love—though I wasn't opposed to it. Later that evening, I spotted a woman standing across the campfire. She had long brown hair, wine-flushed cheeks, and a great smile, and she looked outdoorsy in a no-makeup, natural kind of way. When I found myself standing next to her at the dessert tray, picking at brownies and chocolate chip cookies, I introduced myself. Her name was Hannah Morgan. She was from Utah, played the fiddle, and still used an outdated flip phone. This would be her second summer working at the information desk at the visitor center and leading ranger talks. We chatted a bit more before she told me she had to go home to work on her presentation.

"But you should come to one of my programs some time," she said, giving me a smile as she got ready to leave. "And if you're really good, maybe I'll give you a Junior Ranger badge!"

"It's a deal!"

I watched her as she said goodbye to everyone, handing out hugs over handshakes. When she left the light of the fire, I saw her click on a headlamp, pull a can of bear spray from her pocket, and continue home.

The night ended with Sam, Cody, Zach, and me seated around the fire, using tree stumps for chairs, watching the dying embers. Sam had tossed the cap to the Jack Daniels into the fire, which according to him, meant we had to finish the entire bottle.

It was the third week in May, and the park was still relatively empty.

"When will it pick up?" I asked.

Cody told me not to worry. "It'll be like someone hit a switch, and it will suddenly get busy," he said, like a weatherman spotting a storm front moving in. "Before you know it, thousands of tourists will arrive. Then you'll blink, and your season will be over."

It was hard to believe that quiet night, but Cody was right. Once Memorial Day arrived, the crowds appeared, 9-1-1 calls started popping off, and we didn't slow down again until late September. That's when the bison migrated across Fountain Flats in long, lumbering lines; the grizzlies entered their hyperphagia phase before hibernation, eating everything from seeds, berries, roots, and grasses to dead animals; and the elk went into rut, sounding their mournful bugles over the burnt-orange grasses.

I was in for the time of my life.

A CALL IN THE WILD

MOST PEOPLE IMAGINE an urban or suburban environment when they think of what we call "prehospital emergency medicine." A frantic person dials 9-1-1, and the call is quickly routed to a state-of-the-art call center teeming with computer screens, monitors, and dozens of headset-wearing dispatchers. The caller knows the address he or she is at because it's clearly displayed above the front door, and the dispatcher immediately sends out the nearest fire/EMS agency, which responds in minutes with a team of six—two on the ambulance and four on the fire engine. Everyone on the crew has worked together for years and runs the call like a well-oiled machine. After assessing the patient and providing any initial lifesaving treatment, these strong EMS workers move the patient to the gurney and into the ambulance. There are half a dozen hospitals to choose from, each less than fifteen minutes away, allowing patients to have surgery within the "golden hour," the sixty minutes following an injury during which rapid medical care has the greatest likelihood to prevent morbidity and mortality.

Everyone thinks of this scenario because, since the earliest days of NBC's hit show *Emergency!* in 1972, that's all that's ever been portrayed in television shows and movies.

Of course, the truth of prehospital emergency care in America is vastly different. Millions of people live an hour or more away from their nearest hospital, and over 70 percent of rural EMS agencies rely on volunteers who respond to emergencies with limited personnel, minimal equipment, and long transport times to the hospital.

Consequently, when Cody and Sam debriefed me on EMS operations at Yellowstone, I was given a list of things not to expect: an exact address, good radio communication ability or cell phone service, the same crew to run calls with, a short ETA to the accident scene or hospital, the availability of a medevac helicopter, or even a safe scene.

"No scene safety?" I asked incredulously, "There can't be bison and bears around all the time!"

Cody reminded me over one thousand earthquakes tremored through Yellowstone annually and that I was living in one of the largest supervolcanoes on earth.

"Good point," I chuckled. "But we're all screwed if it blows."

Along with mountains, rivers, jungles, and woods, wilderness medicine also encompasses medical situations underwater, as well as disaster medicine and humanitarian assistance. This emerging field has become immensely popular since people of all ages are embracing far-flung travel and adventure sports, and it promises to keep growing in the future. Many medical schools now offer wilderness medicine fellowships and subspecialties, and as natural disasters continue to occur with greater frequency and impact, it is making "wilderness" medicine applicable even in large cities when resources and utilities are cut off for days. And as I quickly learned in Yellowstone, people didn't leave their medical complaints at home when they traveled to national parks.

I assumed one or two of those urban EMS elements might be missing from a scene, but when Andie Howard from Henderson, Nevada, fell asleep at the wheel two weeks into my season, I discovered they could all be absent at once, to devastating effect.

"Old Faithful EMS, respond to the area around Iron Springs for a vehicle off the roadway." The page sent Sam and me sprinting to the apparatus bay.

Iron Springs was a picnic area forty-five minutes north of Old Faithful on the Grand Loop Highway. However, once we were en route, dispatch informed us the accident had actually occurred twenty minutes earlier because the caller had to drive to get reception. The reporting party thought the accident might have occurred near the Caldera Rim picnic area. But then again, it might have been near Gibbon Meadows. Or maybe it was Tuff Cliff, or Gibbon Falls? Regardless of the exact location, the person was certain that a car had gone off the road into the woods and that the driver was probably dying.

"You asked when the summer season would begin," Sam yelled as we roared out of the apparatus bay. "It's begun!"

The two weeks following the EMS refresher hadn't exactly been slow. As the temperature warmed, campers, RVs, and bus tours had rolled in, and our pagers buzzed with emergency calls. We ran calls for leg cramps, headaches, a hernia, a man with an enlarged prostate who was having difficulty urinating, and one night at 3:30 am, for a man from France who said, "J'ai mal à la poitrine et je suis à bout de souffle," and "J'ai des antécédents de crise cardiaque." We were stumped until his daughter explained, "He has sharp chest pain and is short of breath," so Sam immediately radioed dispatch and said, "Launch an air ambulance."

41

It was the first time I'd ever run a call where a medevac helicopter was requested. Cody assigned me to be the ground contact to help land the helo. "Your job is to ensure the LZ [landing zone] is safe and to update the pilot on wind and visibility," he explained, pointing to a nearby windsock.

Minutes later I radioed the pilot. "We have scattered clouds. Winds are light and variable, and the LZ is secure," I said proudly.

It wasn't long before I ran another medevac call. The very next week, I was the primary patient care provider on a call and requested my first helicopter. An elderly man from Grand Rapids, Michigan, had gone souvenir shopping while his wife took a bath in their room at the Snow Lodge, a modern hotel near Old Faithful. When the man returned half an hour later, he found her unconscious in the bathtub, with first degree burns from the scalding water covering her body. The woman's blood pressure was elevated, and I suspected a stroke. I turned to Sam and said, "Launch a life flight."

I was learning a lot about the EMS operation at Old Faithful—such as when to transport a patient to the Old Faithful Clinic and when to go straight to the hospital and how to set up a rendezvous with an outside agency like Hebgen Basin Fire Department in West Yellowstone, with Madison County Fire Department in Rexburg, or with Grand Teton EMS. Rather than drive the full distance to a hospital, we'd often meet another ambulance service halfway, and hand off our patients there, allowing us return to Yellowstone more quickly. Our transfer points were often gas stations or roadside pullouts; passersby always looked at us strangely, as if some illicit stolen organ operation was going down.

I was also getting my first introduction to long transport times and managing a patient's comfort and pain level over the course of forty-five to ninety minutes, but I was eager to run a call outside in the wild and discover what it felt like when the environment said, "You think it's easy out here? Hold my beer."

This would be my first experience.

As the ambulance sped past the bubbling mud of Fountain Paint Pots, we rounded a corner and encountered a large animal jam. Two dozen bison had formed a defensive line across the two-lane road, stopping traffic in both directions. I shut off the sirens as we approached so as to not send the bison stampeding into the crowd of picture-taking tourists. I chirped the siren as we approached, but the bison barely looked up. I honked, but they'd heard that before. We continued to approach slowly, the grill guard of the ambulance inches from their tawny hides, but they stood firm. We needed to get through. A person was dying. Yet I couldn't drive around them, because the landscape itself was also a fragile protected area. I laid on the horn again.

Nothing.

Suddenly, Sam grabbed the intercom. "Hold on, Lodgepole. I have an idea."

He reminded me that we're in the land of large carnivores. "Grizzlies, wolves, and mountain lions," he said, "who all feast on bison, right?"

Sam handed me the mic. "Let's hear your best mountain lion roar."

I drew in a big breath, depressed the black button, and emitted a scream: *"Ah-ah, ah! Ah-ah, ah! Ah-ah, ah!"*

My scream was high-pitched and pitiful, somewhere between a cougar and Robert Plant's banshee howl at the opening of Led Zeppelin's "Immigrant Song." But it worked.

Baby bison, who didn't know better, skittered off the roadway on thin, coltish legs. The older bison, with thick, rangy coats, didn't quite buy it, but they stepped aside grudgingly as if to honor my attempt.

Once we passed the bison herd, I hit the gas, and dispatch informed us that a ranger was on-scene. The accident had occurred at Iron Springs, where a series of S-shaped curves had a notorious history of slingshotting vehicles forty feet into the woods.

"I have three patients," the ranger announced. "Two with minor wounds and one critical, going in and out of consciousness."

The ranger's name was Chris, and he worked in the Canyon District of the park. Sam and I had never run a call with him before, but we were about to.

"Copy," I replied over the radio. "ETA, twenty minutes."

Sam took the mic from me and requested a helicopter. "We'll land the bird right at the accident scene on the highway."

We'd been driving for half an hour by then, and we still had twenty minutes to go. We'd hardly *reach* our patient within "the golden hour," let alone transport them to definitive care. This meant that instead of receiving a CT scan and life-saving surgery, our patient would likely be succumbing to the "trauma triad of death." Blood loss would decrease tissue perfusion, causing hypothermia and impaired clot formation, which, in turn, would prompt the body to produce lactate and get acidotic. It was all just a scientific way of saying a patient was "circling the drain."

When we arrived on-scene twenty minutes later, Sam and I grabbed a backboard and our BLS bag and started down the steep embankment, sidestepping ankle-deep through small loose stones known as scree. Two of the occupants stood roadside, uninjured. We couldn't see the car, but they pointed and told us it was some-where down the woods.

"Rock!" Sam yelled, as he sent a small boulder rolling toward me. I leapt aside, barely preventing the rock from hitting me in the chest.

As the slope leveled out, we found the car among scattered rocks and broken trees. It was clear that when thirty-four-year-old

Andie Howard dozed off, her Toyota Camry had launched down a steep forty-foot slope, miraculously landing upright. Andie's Camry looked like a dented soda can with four wheels, but the passenger compartment was relatively untouched.

"Spidering on the windshield," Sam noted as we approached.

Lightning-bolt-like fissures in the glass emanated from a circle on the windshield the exact size and shape of a human head.

"She's alert and oriented," Chris announced as we approached. "But she's slow to respond and lethargic."

He'd placed Andie on a nasal cannula and was delivering low-flow oxygen via two small prongs. He'd also wisely covered her with a warm blanket to prevent hypothermia and had placed a cervical collar around her neck. I could see glitter-like shards of glass in her brown hair. A Good Samaritan bystander who'd come over to help crouched in the back seat, holding Andie's head in a neutral, in-line position on the assumption that she likely had a spinal injury.

"ETA on the helicopter, fifteen minutes," dispatch announced over the radio.

We performed a quick assessment and found as Chris had that Andie was alert and oriented but slow to answer and complaining of stomach and shoulder pain. In addition to the head injury, she could likely be bleeding internally. And the shoulder pain? That could be Kehr's sign, referred pain that suggested a potentially life-threatening ruptured spleen.

"We need to get her out of the car and up to the road immediately," Sam said.

We had four rangers and two bystanders on-scene to assist. Chris raised the steering wheel to create space, and Sam moved the driver's seat back and reclined it slightly as I slid a rigid backboard under Andie.

"There's only one way to do this, and it's not going to be comfortable," said Sam.

Like a quarterback calling out the play, he assigned us all positions and then said, "Is anyone not ready?"

Chris and I steadied our grip and remained silent.

"OK, moving on three. One . . . two . . . THREE!"

Using our combined effort, we rotated Andie toward the driver's door, laid her down on the backboard, and then used it to move her out of the car and onto the ground.

Once Andie was belted to the backboard, we lifted her again and moved her toward the road, stepping over downed trees and rocks, carrying the backboard, two on each end and two on the side. Andie was a large woman, and it took all of our collective effort to lift her.

"Stop," I called out, my back muscles spasming.

"Lower," Sam ordered.

We set Andie down, reset, and then lifted once again. But after moving a few feet, we had to rest once more. We could barely lift her on flat ground; between the steep slope and gravity, it was too much.

"What's the plan?" I asked.

Sam said Yellowstone had a technical rescue team, but the members would have to come from all parts of the park. It would take hours. With Andie's lethargy and internal injuries, he didn't think she'd last that long.

So that's it, I thought to myself. *She'll die, and the environment will win this one.*

But just then, Emily and Rachel, Old Faithful's fire officer and district ranger, arrived in a light rescue, a small fire truck loaded with tools like the jaw of life for vehicle extrication. They heard our dilemma and had an idea. "You need raw power. We have an electric winch on the front of this rescue," Rachel said. "We'll attach the winch cable to the top of the backboard. You lift and we'll pull!"

Emily and Rachel's improvised idea was audacious, but hell, we knew it just might work.

I scrambled up the hill, grabbed the cable, and brought it back down to Sam, who secured it to the top of the backboard.

We informed Andie of our extrication plan, but she was too lethargic to understand. We'd perform the rescue maneuver under implied consent.

On Sam's count, we lifted Andie as Emily activated the winch. Then, slowly and methodically, we moved up the hill, taking short breaks every few moments to rest.

Once we arrived at the road, we quickly moved Andie into the ambulance and obtained a set of vital signs as I searched for a site to place an IV. Andie had poor venous access, but after multiple attempts, I was able to place an IV. It was a small, pediatric-sized catheter that looked comical on her thick arms, but I didn't care; we now had venous access through which we could administer pain medication and, if necessary, normal saline to raise her blood pressure.

We heard the rhythmic *whoosh-whoosh-whoosh* of the helicopter approaching. I glanced out the ambulance window to see the bird cresting over the mountains. I'd never been so excited to see a helicopter in my whole life. It descended through the thin clouds and golden sunlight like a heaven-sent angel with a spinning halo of rotor blades.

As I listened to Andie's breath sounds once again, assessing her for a collapsed lung, I could feel the momentum trending in our favor. The location of the accident scene, terrain, and poor access had presented challenges, but we'd adapted and overcome. Andie would now be transported by air to a trauma center, her life would be saved, and the score would be Old Faithful EMS 1, the environment 0.

At least, that was my assumption. But when the flight team hopped out, and the pilot took a look at Andie, he pulled Sam and me aside and said, "We can't fly her. She's over the weight limit."

"What?" I asked. "No!"

The pilot informed me it was a safety issue. Andie weighed too much.

Sam quickly turned to me. "Looks like we'll have to drive her to the hospital."

Sam and I hopped in back of the ambulance, and Chris took the wheel, hightailing it to West Yellowstone. There, we'd transfer care to paramedics with Hebgen Basin Fire Department, who'd transport Andie the rest of the way to the hospital. As we raced around tight curves and bounced over rolling frost heaves, the ambulance pitching and swaying like a small boat on big seas, we gave Andie Fentanyl for pain, saline to maintain her blood pressure, and Zofran for nausea. Once we'd performed most of our paramedic interventions, Sam encouraged me to think of the prolonged transport now as nursing. "We've stabilized her, so now it's all about making a connection with her and ensuring she's warm and comfortable."

Andie's condition didn't really improve on the way to West Yellowstone, but she didn't get worse, so we took it as a win.

"They'll take good care of you, Andie," I said as we moved her into Hebgen Basin's ambulance in the parking lot outside an IMAX theater. "I hope you feel better soon."

After we transferred care, I watched the other ambulance disappear down the road, and I took a seat on our ambulance's bumper, exhausted and sweaty. My first experience running a call in the woods had been messy and muddy. It was challenging and chaotic. Plans changed. Success was never guaranteed, and it had demanded elements of audacity and improvisation.

It was my first wild rescue, and I absolutely loved it.

• • • • • • •

As we drove back to Old Faithful that evening, following the Madison River east before turning south and skirting the dark, shallow splendor that is the Firehole River at dusk, Sam and I debriefed about the call, and he passed along some wilderness EMS pearls of wisdom.

On additional resources: "Order big. Order early. And don't be afraid to cancel extra personnel and apparatus if you don't need them."

On having limited personnel on-scene with you: "Triage your treatment. What needs to be done *right now*, and what can wait? Put bystanders to work."

On the inevitable obstacles that arise: "Learn to compartmentalize, adapt, and overcome."

On having a backup plan: "Nothing is certain out here, so always be asking yourself, 'What's my plan if this doesn't work?'"

On the pace an emergency call should run: "Slow is smooth, and smooth is fast."

And lastly, on the long transport times: "On most calls, the paramedic work is really finished within the first twenty minutes," he said. "After that, it's all about connecting with your patient. Talking is often the best treatment."

I called the Eastern Idaho Regional Medical Center the following day and found out Andie was doing well. She had a mild concussion and a few broken bones but none of the internal injuries we'd been concerned about, and the doctors expected her to make a full recovery.

· · · · · · ·

But not every patient had as good an outcome.

A week later, as a Taiwanese man was seated with his family on the steep hillside behind Grand Prismatic Spring, a dead pine tree with shallow roots toppled over and fell on him, cracking open his skull and leaving only a sunken crater where the left side of his face used to be. Despite Sam, Cody, Backcountry Bill, Emily, and Zach, the law enforcement ranger, all racing to the scene, the man went into traumatic cardiac arrest as they carried him off the hillside. They quickly moved him into the ambulance, but although they valiantly tried to save his life, they were unsuccessful.

It was my day off, so I hadn't been on that call. I'd spent the day driving north to the closest Target, REI, and large grocery store, two and a half hours away in Bozeman, Montana. When I returned, I saw the apparatus bay doors were open at the Emergency Services Building, so I stopped by to help rehab the ambulance.

The patient compartment looked like a murder scene. Gauze, oxygen tubing, suction hoses, exam gloves, plastic wrappers, and IV catheters floated in an inch-deep slurry of blood. I'd been on bad trauma calls before, but this was something else. More like Stephen King's *It* than a typical EMS call.

We all pitched in, using disinfectant spray, towels, and mops to soak up the red stuff. Thirty minutes later, the patient compartment was sparkling. After the rest of the ambulance was clean and restocked, everyone gathered in the conference room for a Critical Stress Incident Debriefing (CISD) to talk about the call: what went well, where they could improve, and—most importantly—if they had any lingering thoughts, feelings, and emotions. It was clear from the comments and quivering voices that it had been a tough call for everyone involved.

As the meeting ended, Emily heard something in the apparatus bay.

Drip . . . drip . . . drip.

It sounded like a leaking faucet, but there wasn't a sink near the ambulance.

Drip . . . drip . . . drip.

Emily went to investigate. "Hey guys," she hollered. "We have an oil leak."

Cody pulled an exam glove from his pocket, knelt, and ran a finger through the viscous fluid.

"Not oil," he said, standing and presenting a dark red fingertip.

"The ambulance is bleeding," Emily declared, aghast.

The patient compartment was clean, but the blood had seeped down tiny cracks and screws holes, penetrating the very core of the ambulance.

Sickened, Sam placed an oil pan underneath the ambulance.

We all left the Emergency Services Building that night in silence, badly shaken. I was just about to walk to the eight-plex when Cody tossed me the keys to another rig: Yellowstone's newest ambulance, Old Faithful No. 1.

"We staff two ambulances here," he explained. "And the second one is all yours."

"OF1" was a badass rig. It was a Type-1, box-style ambulance that sat on a Ford F-350 Chassis with four thick tires and had a big silver grille guard to protect against any unfortunate encounters with large, hooved ungulates like bison, deer, or elk.

"Thanks," I replied, catching the keys. "But why?"

Cody explained that OF1 was now mine to drive to and from work each day and to any emergency calls in between. Technically, I was only scheduled for eight hours a day, but the unwritten rule was that I ought to take any late-night page-outs if I wanted to earn rehire status, guaranteeing me employment in future seasons.

"Don't worry," I said quickly, "I'll take all the night calls."

By handing over the keys, Cody was saying that my field training was officially over. "Nice work, Lodgepole."

After Cody left, I hopped in OF1 and drove around the government area, saying hello and waving to everyone.

"Nice ride!" yelled Will, the VIP, as he sat enjoying the sunshine with Sarah in front of their RV.

Like the ranger at Yosemite with his rattling snow chains who'd first inspired me to pursue a job with the NPS, I was now a shepherd, looking after my flock. Some of the people in the government area I knew; others I didn't; but no matter—without the slightest hesitation, I would gladly risk my life to save theirs.

After the government area, I drove the ambulance to check out some hot springs at Biscuit Basin and Black Sand Basin. I was like a just-licensed sixteen-year-old showing off his new ride, but as I parked in front of my apartment that night, I had a worrisome realization: no one was riding with me, and I found the prospect of running an emergency entirely by myself downright terrifying.

ALONE ON THE AMBULANCE

THIS SHOULD BE THE PART IN THE STORY when I tell you about my partner on the ambulance—how we spend hours together saving lives and, in between calls, have witty banter about relationships, sports, and politics. My coworkers in Los Angeles had been a rotating eclectic cast of characters. Miguel liked to floor it down Figueroa, swerving in and out of traffic, while making Space Invaders sounds with the sirens and yelling, "Drive it like you stole it!"

Nate was a wannabe ladies' man who got tendonitis in his thumb after spending hours right-swiping to "like" thousands of women on his various dating apps.

Rachel declared me her "Instagram work husband" and always had me snapping pictures of her around the ambulance that she could post on social media, and Cliff enjoyed spending his down time in the back of the ambulance, sleeping on the same gurney we had just cleaned of every kind of fluid that could flow forth from a human being.

I was excited to work with a partner at Yellowstone, but I quickly learned that on most days, I'd be alone on the ambulance. Old Faithful had a unique response model: I'd drive the "ambo" to an emergency call solo and meet law enforcement rangers who were also trained as EMTs, park medics, and paramedics. Then, when transporting the patient to the Old Faithful clinic or the hospital, an LE ranger—or Backcountry Bill, Emily, Will, or another VIP—would hop in to drive.

It's no surprise that I found racing to an emergency scene alone in the ambulance scary as hell, but I quickly learned that the system worked. When Mary from Coeur d'Alene had a sudden onset of abdominal cramping on the Old Faithful boardwalk and knew with heartbreaking certainty that she was having another miscarriage, I pulled up to find that Zach had gotten there first, had already ruled out any life-threatening bleeding, and had taken a set of vital signs, ensuring Mary had received immediate care despite my delayed arrival in the ambulance.

The system worked when Bill from Ottawa had a seizure while driving near Lewis Lake and launched his car into the woods, and when Edith, visiting from England, woke up at 4:00 AM with a wild and irregular heartbeat and said she hadn't been sleeping or eating well since her husband of forty years died unexpectedly three months earlier. The system worked when Wilbur from Maine was scuba diving in the Firehole River, and his buddies found him floating, unresponsive and blue, and when a motorcyclist took a blind corner wide near West Thumb Geyser Basin and joined the bugs in the front grill of a Ford F-350. It worked when a four-year-old Chinese boy's eyes rolled into the back of his head, and his body convulsed in a life-threatening seizure outside the Old Faithful Inn. During each of those calls,

I arrived to find an LE ranger had gotten on-scene ahead of me, performed a great assessment, and provided initial life-saving treatment.

The system worked . . . until it didn't.

It was 2:00 PM one Thursday afternoon when I was dispatched to the Old Faithful Visitor Center to treat a pediatric patient who'd fallen, and I learned that no LE rangers were available to respond. They were spread out all around the park, doing LE ranger things like preventing people from walking across fragile geyser basins, enforcing food storage rules so bears didn't get into coolers, assisting people locked out of their cars, nabbing out-of-bounds campers, and responding to minor fender benders.

As I pulled up to the curb outside of the visitor center, I saw Hannah, the interpretation ranger I'd met at the barbecue, waving me down. Just a few hours earlier, I'd stood on the boardwalk at Castle Geyser with a half dozen families, listening to her ranger-led program on Old Faithful's unique geology and hydrothermal features. I loved that Hannah was so passionate about rocks, steam, and fault lines, but I was only half listening. Most of my attention was focused on her bright smile, free spirit, and the wonderful rapport she had with the families and tourists. Hannah had the kind of childlike connection to the natural world I could only hope to share one day.

After the presentation, I'd walked her back to the information desk and asked her to get together. "We could grab dinner at the Old Faithful Inn one night?"

Hannah agreed. "But the Inn is so expensive," she said, pondering other options for a moment before suddenly lighting up with excitement. "It's a full moon on Thursday! How about we make dinner at your place and then take some wine out to the geyser boardwalk?"

"Perfect!" I replied. "I have cabernet and to-go coffee mugs!"

When I'd left Hannah after that, we'd both walked away happy and excited. But now, as I parked OF1 curbside, she looked very worried.

A young girl sat crying and cradling her right forearm. I jumped out of the ambulance to find the girl's parents arguing with thick Atlantic City accents.

"Way to watch your daughter!"

"Whatever. Don't talk to me like that!"

"We're not in the city! You need to keep a better eye on her!"

I grabbed the BLS bag from the back of the ambulance and hurried over, hoping this call would go better than the first time I'd showed up on-scene solo, for a concession worker named Taryn who'd fainted at the employee dorm and then crawled into the hallway to call 9-1-1.

When I'd arrived on that scene and realized no other rangers were responding, I'd freaked out. I was horribly out of breath, and my patient assessment was all over the place. "What happened? Do you have any allergies? What's your home address?"

Taryn was a nineteen-year-old girl from Iowa, wearing a blue sweat suit that said "Pink." She worked in the cafeteria at the Old Faithful Lodge and had been complaining of a bad headache and sore throat for the last twenty-four hours. She'd called in sick that morning and was in the bathroom, about to get some water, when she suddenly felt like she was going to faint and lowered herself to the floor.

"Got it," I said, writing the information down on the palm of my exam glove, my hand shaking with nerves.

I managed to check her heart rate, blood pressure, respiratory rate, and blood sugar, determined that she hadn't suffered any trauma, and confirmed she wanted to be transported to the clinic. But I was so embarrassed about my rambling patient assessment, nerves, and inability to connect with Taryn that I could barely face her. Instead, I hid behind my equipment—gazing intently at the cardiac monitor to hide my shame—and just kept rechecking her vital signs.

Eventually, Emily showed up to drive the ambulance, and we transported Taryn to the clinic, but I continued to feel awful. I could forgive myself for being nervous, but it was inexcusable that I had failed to comfort this nineteen-year-old girl who was away from home for the first time, sick, and scared. I'd been entirely focused on my own worries and fears, when all of my attention should've been squarely on her.

I remembered that botched call as I hurried alone toward the upset little girl in front of the visitor center. As I set down the BLS bag, Hannah said, "This is McKenzie, and she may have broken her arm."

"Hi McKenzie," I said, taking a knee so I wouldn't be talking down to her. "Can you tell me what hurts today?"

McKenzie was a freckled girl wearing a Taylor Swift T-shirt. I quickly learned she had been walking atop a fallen spruce tree, like it was a balance beam, and fell off, landing on her outstretched arm. She didn't lose consciousness, but her right forearm had an obvious deformity—suggesting that she'd broken her radius and ulna.

"How would you rate the pain?"

McKenzie mumbled something, but I could barely hear her over her parents' bickering.

"Don't talk to me like that!"

"Aww forget about it! Go get a drink of water and cool off!"

I handed McKenzie's dad my notebook and gave him a task to distract him. "Can you please write down her name, address, and date of birth?"

"Mom," I said, turning, "I need you stabilize her arm so I can splint it."

With the parents now occupied, I turned my attention to McKenzie. *Nothing exists in the world but her. She has my full attention.* I reminded her of my name and that I was there to help. I asked to see her arm. McKenzie removed the blanket over her arm and began crying again. I wanted to check her heart rate and blood pressure, but I knew vital signs could wait. Numbers were nice, but they never saved a life, nor directly treated a patient's pain. I decided to first splint McKenzie's arm. As I veered off the typical patient assessment algorithm—improvising for the first time—I felt a rush of excitement.

I delicately placed her arm into a soft splint, secured it with an ACE wrap, and then immobilized her arm by creating a sling and swathe with two fabric triangle bandages.

"How's your pain now?"

"Better, but it still hurts," she said.

After splinting her arm, Hannah and I assisted her onto the gurney.

I knew this would be a transfer to the hospital. Once her mom told me Grand Teton was their next destination, I asked dispatch to page-out for a driver and arrange a rendezvous with Grand Teton EMS to take McKenzie to St. John's Medical Center in Jackson Hole.

Next, we loaded McKenzie into the ambulance. As the back doors closed, I cranked the AC and felt a positive momentum building. I was expecting the call to go south at any moment, but surprisingly, despite me being alone on scene, everything was going according to plan: I'd dealt with the bickering parents, comforted McKenzie, splinted her arm, and removed her from the hot environment and public setting. I was now back in my office, the ambulance.

Once in the ambulance, I had a treatment plan in mind and followed it in rapid succession: I checked McKenzie's vital signs—which came back within normal limits—and, because of her young age, phoned medical control to verify my dose of the narcotic, fentanyl. Next, I placed a 22-gauge IV catheter in her arm, hung a 500-milliliter bag of normal saline and administered fifteen micrograms of fentanyl, starting the dose on the low end to see how she tolerated the medicine.

As I finished pushing the medication, dispatch informed me that there were still no rangers available but that Will, the retired VIP, was en route from the government area. He arrived minutes later in jeans, white T-shirt, and a baseball cap with the Volunteers-in-Parks logo. I introduced Will to McKenzie and her family, and, like everyone, they immediately loved him.

McKenzie's mom hopped in back with McKenzie and me. Her dad and brother would pack up their belongings at the Snow Lodge and drive their rental car to meet McKenzie and her mother in Jackson Hole.

We began transport south toward the Colter Bay District of Grand Teton National Park, ninety minutes away. My work was cut out for me during the long transport: I had to manage McKenzie's pain over the long and bumpy transport but not give her too much fentanyl, which could drop her blood pressure and heart rate. Most importantly, I needed to make that connection with McKenzie and her mom. My goal was to ensure the call had a good outcome and to transform their terrible day at Yellowstone into a fun family memory. As we passed West Elbow junction, I gave McKenzie a second dose of fentanyl and replaced her ice pack.

To get the girl's attention off her injury, I asked about her favorite sport.

"Gymnastics!" she exclaimed before telling me all about her floor and vault routines.

McKenzie's mom leaned in to show me a cell phone video of her daughter. "I could talk your ear off about how proud I am of her."

We also talked about McKenzie's favorite food (pizza), McKenzie's favorite movie (Frozen), and the best part of Yellowstone (swimming in the Boiling River). By the time we arrived in Colter Bay, the kind of alchemy I'd been hoping for had occurred. The call had begun as a tragic and terrible day, but now it had been transformed into a story about McKenzie's adventure in the ambulance that ended on a good note.

Before we transferred her to Grand Teton EMS, McKenzie's mom snapped cell phone pictures of her daughter standing outside the ambulance.

"Aww, get in there with her," Mom said, gesturing with white-tipped French manicured nails.

It wasn't just McKenzie who had overcome something that day. As Will and I drove home through the John D. Rockefeller Jr. Memorial Parkway, which connects Grand Teton and Yellowstone, it dawned on me that I'd just run an emergency call for a pediatric patient requiring advanced life support with no other medical providers. The scene management, patient assessment, splinting, vital signs, medical control, IV, pain medication, and paperwork—I'd done it all alone.

Solo calls had now happened to me twice, and the busy summer season had just begun. I was pleased with my performance—especially after the earlier botched call at the employee dorm—but I couldn't help feeling unease about being alone in the ambulance. It was highly unusual—the sort of thing that would never happen in an urban environment.

"What if I'm by myself, and the patient is critical?" I asked Sam and Cody later that night as we sat staring at the dying embers of a campfire.

"Then you're by yourself with a dying patient," Sam said, standing to leave.

"And then?"

Cody swirled the ice in his whiskey glass. "It's sink or swim."

7

CONCESSIONAIRE CRAZINESS

THE MOCK PATIENTS we practiced emergency scenarios on during the EMS refresher all had one chief drawback: they were always found lying at the center of warm, well-lit rooms, and they were eager to answer questions and help with your assessment. They were nothing like the drunk concession employee we struggled to treat one night at Laurel Dorm, a guy who both happened to have chest pain *and* wanted to kick our asses.

It was after midnight on a Monday when Sam, Emily, Zach, and I responded to an emergency in the filthy carpeted hallway of Laurel Dorm for Davy, a fifty-four-year-old intoxicated man from Slidell, Louisiana.

Davy was an unkempt-looking man with a scraggly gray beard, wild bloodshot eyes, and yellow teeth, who admitted to drinking a lot of beer and liquor that evening. It would've been a fairly straightforward call for chest pain if he hadn't also been combative and intoxicated.

"Davy," I said, holding the cardiac monitor. "I need to perform an EKG to make sure you're not having a heart attack."

"Get away from me!" Davy yelled, flailing his arms and crawling away.

"Davy, come back!" I hollered.

"Screw all of you!"

It was the first big call I led after finishing my field training, and I wanted to make a good impression on Sam, Cody, and the others, but Davy was making it very difficult.

Zach stepped in front of him. "Sir, please hold still."

Sam placed four tablets of baby aspirin into Davy's fist and told him to chew them up, but Davy hurled them across the room. "Get away!"

"If you have chest pain, you need an aspirin," I said, grabbing four more tablets.

Since Davy was drunk and not answering our questions appropriately, I also deemed him unfit to refuse care.

"I need you to chew up these baby aspirins."

"Like hell I will!"

Suddenly Davy's whole body went limp.

"Davy?" I asked, nudging his shoulder. "Wake up!"

I turned to Sam, Cody, and the others. "I think he might've gone into cardiac arrest!" I announced, checking his pulse.

In hindsight, I should've known right away that the call had the potential to be difficult because it came in after midnight. For an intoxicated person. At Laurel Dorm. The dilapidated structure was proof that every area—even a UNESCO World Heritage site like Yellowstone—had a bad part of town. Built in 1926, Laurel was a two-story decaying wooden structure where concession employees were packed in like sardines. The teetering abode had small rooms, thin walls, community bathrooms with cold showers, and, for years, a reputation for giving park rangers trouble. Maybe the high call volume was due to the fact that the youngest workers were often housed in Laurel, where they had easy access to alcohol, even though many of them were underage. Or perhaps it was because the dorm also housed the oldest concession workers, like Davy, who didn't fit in anywhere else. Or maybe it was just because Laurel Dorm was situated on the sinking land adjacent to a thermal area, and there was just something about those gas emissions that messed with everyone's mind.

"Always lock the ambulance doors when you respond to Laurel," Cody had told me during a familiarization tour of the area, "and keep your head on a swivel."

Davy and a few other of Laurel's inhabitants lived—according to one worker—"a life of perpetual work, exhaustion, and ritual drinking." They were employed by the park's contracted concessionaire, a non-NPS entity, which operated many of the restaurants, hotels, stores, and campgrounds in Yellowstone and other national parks throughout the country. Now I'm sure the concessionaire hires many healthy, sober, and law-abiding citizens, but given that I worked in the Visitor and Resource Protection Division, I didn't encounter many of them.

"You only see the deviant ones!" declared Drew, a security guard from Nebraska who was perpetually chewing tobacco.

According to Drew, the concessionaire hired double their staffing needs each summer because they knew they would fire half of them. Those concession employees that made it through the summer season attended a "survivor's party" where they celebrated a summer of drinking by indulging in even more alcoholic beverages.

However, that night in Laurel Dorm, I didn't much care about Davy's background. My job as a paramedic was to provide nonjudgmental, compassionate care and, right then, that began with determining if he had a pulse.

I couldn't find one, so I looked over at Zach. "Begin chest compressions."

Zach dropped to his knees and positioned himself to start CPR, but suddenly Davy woke up with a jolt and resumed shouting and flailing. "Git th' hell away from me!"

"Time to make decisions," said Sam, motioning to his watch. "What's the plan?"

We'd been on-scene for twenty minutes. I needed to determine if Davy needed to get to a hospital or simply sober up in jail.

Davy's blood pressure and pulse were elevated, suggesting his heart was in distress, and he had chest pain. "Order big. Order early. And don't be afraid to cancel extra personnel and apparatus if you don't need them," Sam had said when we'd used the winch cable at Iron Springs. But Davy was also drunk as hell and wouldn't let us start an IV, administer medication, or perform an EKG to take a detailed look at his heart. *He should go to jail for public intox!* Then again, he did have that brief moment when he appeared to lose a pulse.

"So, which is it?" Sam demanded.

I asked Davy if his chest still hurt.

"Awww it hurts *r-e-a-l* bad," he slurred like a bad actor.

I decided to sway on the side of caution and instructed Zach to page-out for the clinic staff and request a helicopter.

"Copy," he replied, walking down the hall and summoning dispatch on the radio.

As we moved Davy onto the gurney and into the ambulance, his whole affect changed, and he resembled a mischievous little kid who'd gotten away with something. The friendly drunk replaced the boisterous and belligerent one.

As Emily and I continued our assessment, he began hitting on her. "Hey, baby," he said, blinking bloodshot eyes and massaging his scraggly beard. "You're kinda cute!"

As we made the short drive to the clinic, I felt the need to justify my decision to call for the clinic staff and helicopter. "He has chest pain," I began. "How many drunk patients complain of that?"

"A lot," Sam replied. "They have *incarceritis*, don't want to go to jail."

I kicked myself, fearing Zach, Sam, and Cody had lost confidence in me as a patient care provider.

We arrived at the clinic to find Anne, the physician's assistant, and Jessica, the nurse, waiting for us. They looked half asleep with blue scrubs thrown over pajamas.

"You got a boyfriend?" Davy asked Emily as we transferred him to the clinic bed.

"Yes, sir," she replied, "and he carries a gun."

Davy turned his attention to Jessica. "Hey, beautiful," he said with whiskey breath. "You single?"

"Nope," she said, presenting her left index finger. "Married."

Whether he was sobering up or just trying to impress Emily and Jessica, Davy finally allowed us to start an IV and perform a 12-lead EKG. His heart rhythm appeared normal, but he still needed to go the hospital to get his blood work done and rule out a heart attack.

By the time the helicopter landed outside at 1:00 am, Davy was feeling better.

"I need a cigarette before we go!" he pleaded as we wheeled him to the helicopter. "Please!"

"You're complaining of chest pain," I reminded him. "No!"

As we loaded Davy onto the helicopter, he turned his attention to the flight nurse. "Hey, baby," he said, shaking her hand. "You got a boyfriend?"

The helicopter launched moments later, rising into the night like an electric insect. When it disappeared over the surrounding mountains, bound for the cardiac floor at Eastern Idaho Regional Medical Center, I thanked the clinic staff for their response and turned off the green helipad lights.

"Nice work, Lodgepole," Sam said, smiling. "I think you just flew out a drunk guy."

I second-guessed my decision to fly Davy for the next few days. I felt stupid and embarrassed, and I could only imagine the stories my friends would tell at future EMS refreshers: "And one time, this paramedic from Los Angeles ordered a life flight helicopter for a drunk guy." Along with this, I also felt bad for Davy. A helicopter bill can easily exceed $20 thousand. Did he have insurance? Would his company pay for the flight if it wasn't medically necessary?

Fortunately, I got my answer the following week as I held the door to the Old Faithful Ranger Station for a man with yellow teeth who wore a stained white t-shirt under blue overalls.

"Thank you," he muttered, his breath smelling of cigarettes.

"Davy?" I asked.

Davy looked up, startled. "Do I know you?"

I informed Davy I was the paramedic who'd helped him the other night. "I treated you and called the helicopter."

I expected an outpouring of emotion from Davy for saving his life.

"Huh?" Davy asked. "What are you talking about?"

That was when I realized that, indeed, I flew out a drunk guy.

"If you'll excuse me, I have an appointment at the clinic," Davy said, pushing past me. "Have to follow up on a few stents I just got."

A drunk guy having a heart attack.

BUCKET LIST

TYPICAL DAYS DON'T EXIST when you work in a national park. Every morning as I stepped out of my apartment and called "in-service" over the radio, I never knew if the dispatcher would send me on a 9-1-1 call, a patient transfer from the Old Faithful Clinic to one of the regional hospitals, a search for a lost child, or a bison jam where I'd be directing traffic. Or dispatch could tell me to help in "hazing" (i.e., moving) a grizzly bear separating parents and their children on the path leading to Morning Glory, rescuing a dog from a hot parked car, or trapping an angry pine marten that had taken up residence in the dry storage of the kitchen at the Old Faithful Inn.

In between those requests, I kept the EMS program running by refilling oxygen bottles, inventorying our medications and equipment, washing the ambulance, teaching continuing education classes, and repairing the training mannequins. The arms and legs of "Mannequin Mike," "Mini Mannequin," and "Premature Man-nequin Anne" were always falling off, making the training room look like the gruesome scene of a multiple amputation.

Once I completed these tasks, I'd don my flat hat and take a little tour of the Old Faithful District. I'd stroll to the clinic to say hello to Anne and Jessica and then wander across the hall to the permit office to check in with Backcountry Bill, Will, and Sarah. They were always busy handing out camping permits and telling guests things like, "Sorry, there are no hot showers at backcountry sites," and "It's bear spray, not bug repellant, so please don't douse your kids."

Next, I'd drive OF1 across the parking lot to visit Hannah at the visitor center. I always made it a point to say hello to her every day I worked. We'd been friends since I'd attended her talk that afternoon in early June, and we spent our days off hiking or taking a scenic float on the Yellowstone River through Gar-diner, Montana. On many nights, we'd wander the Upper Geyser Basin boardwalks, sipping wine. It was there, under a full moon and beside splashing geysers, that we often discussed future plans, and I told her about my dream to work as a firefighter paramedic in Los Angeles. One night, my musing was interrupted by a long, mournful howl.

"Holy shit, a wolf!" I said, pulling away.

"Coyote," Hannah replied calmly.

We returned to our conversation, only to hear a chorus of yips and barks sounding from all directions.

"We better leave," I said, grabbing my bear spray.

"Yeah," Hannah added, seriously. "We might be surrounded!"

After saying hello to her at the visitor center, I'd wander the boardwalks around Old Faithful and meet visitors from all over the world—Australia, India, England, South Africa, Thailand, Peru, and—of course—from all over the United States. I loved talking with them and really seeing the national park come alive in their eyes, in their clicking cameras and bright smiles. My role was that of a host—*Welcome to Yellowstone!*—so I'd shake their hands, find out where they were visiting from, and answer their questions, which ranged from logistical to comical, to scientific or historical: *Where are the bathrooms? What time will Old Faithful erupt? Are those bright colors around hot springs really heat-loving bacteria? Where are the yellow stones? When do the deer turn into elk? Where's the switch that turns on Old Faithful? What time do you put the bison back into their cages? Where's Half Dome?*

"I'm sorry," I'd reply. "Half Dome is in Yosemite, which is located in California."

People were always getting Yellowstone confused with the other Y park.

One woman followed up by asking for directions to Vernal Falls.

"That's in Yosemite too," I told her. "But we have the Grand Canyon of Yellowstone. It's absolutely amazing."

"Whatever," said the woman, storming away. I had the feeling she was probably the type who gave national parks a one-star review on Yelp.

I was returning to the ambulance on a Saturday after one such stroll when I spotted a large elderly man seated on the hot pavement next to his car. A strawberry-like abrasion covered his right elbow, and his wife stood next to him, looking worried. I knew immediately that he'd fallen.

I rushed over to help. "Sir, are you OK?"

"I was trying to move from the car to my wheelchair but missed," he explained.

Arthur was an eighty-year-old man from Mesa, Arizona, who wore a ballcap decorated with the ribbon from the National

Defense Service Medal and had "United States Veteran" inscribed with bold yellow stitching.

"I'm too weak to lift him on my own," added his wife, a thin woman named Marilyn.

I quickly assessed that Arthur didn't so much fall as he'd slumped to the ground, and he denied any significant injuries. "I don't need medical treatment," Arthur confessed, "but I'd greatly appreciate some help getting back in my wheelchair. I've been waiting my whole life to see Old Faithful!"

Due to his large size, I couldn't lift Arthur on my own, and no LE rangers were immediately available, so I radioed the visitor center to send out two interps. Moments later, Hannah hurried out with Deb, a red-headed woman in her fifties from Worcester, Massachusetts, with a thick New England accent.

Using our combined strength, we assisted Arthur to his feet and slowly sat him down.

I thanked Hannah and Deb and then assumed my place behind the wheelchair. "Where to?"

Marilyn said not to trouble myself. "I can push him."

I said it would be my honor to help.

"To the boardwalk then," Marilyn replied, pulling a camera from her coat pocket. "It's always been our dream to see the Queen of Geysers."

Arthur said he hadn't thought he'd ever make it. "But here I am." The tone of his voice indicated he may have gone through many ambulance rides, urgent surgeries, and long recoveries.

Yellowstone hosted every type of tourist—families, road bikers, motorcycle gangs, backpackers, hitchhikers, geyser gazers, wolf-watchers, newlyweds, and the recently separated. "Just Divorced!" I saw written in bar soap on the back window of a Honda Accord one afternoon. "YOLOstone!"

There was also a special subset of visitors who, like Arthur, wanted to experience the wonders of Yellowstone for the first, and last, time.

Like anyone on vacation, the bucket listers sought freedom from their normal schedule and the S-M-T-W-T-F-S plastic pill organizers that ruled their lives back home. But frequently, this meant they'd stop taking their prescribed medications that prevented clots, maintained glucose levels, or reduced blood pressure. Most often, they'd stop taking the water pill that made them pee frequently because doing so would be such a hassle on those long bus tours. These bucket listers would arrive at Old Faithful, where sleep loss, preexisting conditions, dehydration, and altitude would hit them like a hammer. The 9-1-1 calls for shortness of breath, chest pain, dizziness, or grossly swollen ankles caused by congestive heart failure would inevitably come in.

You shouldn't be here! I thought to myself one night at 2:45 AM when a sixty-year-old obese man named Wilbur from Clayton, Georgia, told me in his southern drawl that his medical history included "two double bypass surgeries, seven heart attacks, five stents in ma' heart, three stents in ma' legs, chronic back pain, and diabetes." And he smoked a pack of Marlboro Reds every day.

Wilbur had called 9-1-1 when he woke up with heart palpitations and chest pain. When I learned of his medical history and spotted his abnormal EKG—along with ***Acute MI Suspected***—I immediately paged-out the clinic staff and requested a medevac, because it appeared he was having a myocardial infarction (MI), or heart attack.

We stabilized Wilbur and loaded him in the helo, but as it rose from the helipad, he had a panic attack.

"Git me off this fuckin' thang!" he yelled, thrashing and nearly crashing the bird. "I'm gunna die!"

We ended up transporting Wilbur by ambulance to Madison Memorial Hospital in Rexburg, Idaho, via a rendezvous with Hebgen Basin Fire Department. At the hospital, the cardiologist discovered Wilbur wasn't having a heart attack; his abnormal-looking EKG was his "new normal" after having so many cardiac incidents in the past. Given his extensive medical history and the fact that Old Faithful sat well over a mile above sea level, the doctor told Wilbur not to return to Yellowstone.

So what did he do?

The moment he was discharged, Wilbur and his wife immediately drove back to Old Faithful where he, once again, called 9-1-1 at 2:00 AM for chest pain, shortness of breath, and palpitations. Luckily, I was off and not in the area, but I heard all about it from Sam, Cody, and Zach.

I had never quite understood why these elderly people routinely risked their lives to visit Yellowstone, defying their doctor's orders with all the urgency of a Pacific salmon swimming upstream. I had assumed the old and infirm were just being stubborn. But everything changed when I encountered an older Japanese man named Riku one afternoon in the clinic. He had a pulsating mass in his stomach, suggestive of an abdominal aortic aneurysm (AAA), and the EKG monitor showed signs of an acute MI. Both the AAA and acute MI could kill Riku, so naturally we wanted to do everything we could to save him. But when we proposed our treatment plan of a full workup and medevac helicopter, Riku said something softly in Japanese and pointed an ancient finger toward the door.

"He wants to be with his family," his daughter, herself a physician, translated. "And be outside."

"But he could die at any moment," pleaded Anne, the physician assistant.

Riku nodded with twinkling eyes.

"He knows," his daughter announced. "He wants to see the dancing geysers."

I'd never encountered anyone like Riku. Old age and disease had ravaged his body, and yet his eyes and spirit appeared ageless. He was adamant about refusing treatment, so he and his family signed the discharge papers, and we assisted him to his car in a wheelchair.

I was distraught after the family left, and I didn't understand Riku's decision until a few weeks later, when I read Dr. Atul Gawande's classic, *Being Mortal*. In the book, he maintains that our job in medicine is not to prolong life at all costs but rather to support well-being and the reasons people have for living. As medical professionals working with Western medicine, there is always another intervention we can perform, but that doesn't always mean we should do it. What creates meaning in a patient's life? How does the patient find purpose? "Understanding the finitude of one's life could be a gift," Dr. Gawande writes. "Our ultimate goal, after all, is not a good death but a good life to the very end."

After meeting Riku and reading *Being Mortal*, I never questioned the bucket listers again or rolled my eyes when the alarm tones sounded for someone with swollen ankles or shortness of breath at 2:00 AM. There was a life-affirming defiance of death in their decision to visit Yellowstone, and I came to love them for it.

· · · · · · ·

As I pushed Arthur up the sloping sidewalk between the visitor center and the Old Faithful Inn that afternoon, he and Marilyn teared up when they saw the Upper Geyser Basin for the very first time.

Suddenly, I noticed a spring bubbling in the far distance.

"Look!" I exclaimed. "The indicator is going off! Beehive is about to blow!"

"Excuse me?" said Arthur.

I quickly explained that the bubbling spring indicated that my favorite geyser—named Beehive—was about to erupt. I was going to tell them how Beehive was higher than Old Faithful and shot water through its vent faster than the speed of sound, but the geyser spoke for itself, launching a torrent of water and a fine veil of rainbow mist two hundred feet in the air with a jet engine roar.

"Wow," Arthur exclaimed joyously, tearing up again and reaching for Marilyn's hand.

The geothermal show continued for a few more minutes, and then as Beehive died down, Arthur looked over at me. "That was everything," he says, his voice trembling. "Thank you."

• • • • • • •

Old Faithful wasn't scheduled to erupt for an hour, and Arthur and Marilyn wanted to grab lunch, so I gave them the phone number for dispatch and told them to call when they were ready to leave. "I'll be just across the parking lot at the ranger station," I said, pointing. "Give us a call, and we'll help you back into your car."

When dispatch summoned me an hour later, I grabbed Zach and Backcountry Bill, and we drove over in OF1. But when we arrived, we discovered Arthur in the front passenger seat and Marilyn behind the wheel.

"I'm sorry I wasn't here to help," I said, hurrying up.

"Don't worry," Arthur replied. "You were."

I asked Arthur how he enjoyed Old Faithful, and he gave me a thumbs-up. "But not as impressive as Beehive."

When Marilyn mentioned they were driving to Grand Teton to spend the night at Jackson Lake Lodge, I offered to call the Teton rangers. After all, along with being a super nice guy, Arthur was a veteran who served our country. It was the least I could do.

Marilyn told me not to worry. They'd find a way.

"We always do," added Arthur softly.

"OK," I replied, suddenly sad.

The moment of goodbye arrived, and I knew I'd never see Arthur in this world again. Sure, I'd only met him hours earlier, but we'd watched Beehive erupt together. We'd shared the same sense of awe, and that moment would be ours forever.

"Safe travels, sir." I said, shaking his hand.

The gesture seemed too formal, so I leaned in for a hug.

"Take care, old boy," Arthur replied.

Once Arthur and Marilyn left, I dropped off Zach and Backcountry Bill at the ranger station and then drove north to Biscuit Basin, feeling at once both heartbroken and healed.

Later, as I wandered Biscuit Basin's wooden boardwalk, white steam rose from sapphire pools, dark ravens poked for leftovers on picnic tables, and at twilight, a bull bison crossed the Firehole River.

Yellowstone was always reminding me that life was beautifully sweet but also fragile and fleeting.

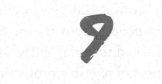

JOB SECURITY

A TWO-THOUSAND-POUND BISON with sharp horns loitered beside the asphalt path near Castle Geyser.

Most people know to keep a good distance between themselves and the largest land-dwelling mammal in North America—which can run more than thirty miles per hour and jump five feet vertically—but some tourists check their common sense at the Roosevelt Arch leading into Yellowstone. So there I was in my green and gray uniform and flat hat making sure everyone stayed twenty-five yards away.

"Back up!" I shouted to a crowd of a half dozen smartphone- and tablet-toting visitors.

"Can we pet the bison?" a man asked.

"No."

A teenage girl hurried over. "Can I take a selfie with one?"

"Not unless you want a ride in my ambulance."

Will, dressed in his volunteer uniform, worked the crowd on the far side of the path. "Ma'am, please move back," he said in his polite, southern drawl. "Sir, kindly step away from the bison."

It wasn't the first time I'd found myself in this position. When I'd first arrived at Old Faithful, I'd assumed my primary duty would be to protect the people from the park's many dangers: bears, wolves, hot springs, and towering cliffs. However, I quickly realized I would spend most of my time protecting the four-legged creatures from the two-legged ones. One incident with a grizzly bear illustrated this reversal perfectly.

It was a busy afternoon in August, and hundreds of tourists had gathered around the Old Faithful geyser when the bruin appeared.

I'd just reunited a lost four-year-old with her family on the boardwalk when I heard Zach announce over the radio, "All units be advised; we have a grizzly running from the ranger station toward the visitor center."

I said a quick goodbye to the family, hopped in the ambulance, and pulled out.

The area was crowded with families and tourists streaming toward the boardwalk to watch the legendary geyser erupt. Suddenly I saw the bear, a juvenile grizzly with a tawny brown coat, sprinting through the parking lot with Zach trailing fifty yards behind in his patrol car.

"OF1," he said over the radio, spotting me. "Pull forward and see if you can use the ambulance to change the bear's direction."

"Copy," I replied, speeding up.

As I approached the bear, I hoped he'd veer left and run back into the woods on the other side of the parking lot, but when he saw the ambulance, he increased his pace and disappeared around the visitor center. I couldn't see what happened next, but I heard screams as tourists scattered.

Zach drove up and over the curb and followed the bear. I turned the ambulance around and sped back to the Old Faithful Lodge, the closest access point to the boardwalk. That would be the easiest spot to pick up the multiple patients—or fatalities—I assumed we'd have. I expected the victims to have bone-deep marks on their forearms from trying to fight back and possibly even puncture wounds to the head. The official cause of death? Blunt force trauma and bleeding out, after encountering North America's apex predator, *Ursus arctos horribilis.*

That was the scene I prepared for as I parked, but when I looked up, I saw the bear had climbed a tree and was now staring down at a hysterical mob of tourists, all jostling closer to take photos.

"Everybody back!" Zach yelled, jumping out of his car and waving his arms at the swelling tide of tourists.

I donned my flat hat, grabbed a fluorescent traffic vest and a can of bear spray, and hurried over to help.

The bear climbed higher in the tree, the branches bending underneath his weight. North America's apex predator had become prey. I realized most of the incidents involving humans and wildlife these days weren't caused by the wildlife.

For instance, there were five bison gorings during my time at Yellowstone. The first occurred in May, when a Taiwanese girl was gored in the buttocks while attempting to take a selfie.

A sixty-two-year-old man from Australia was the second victim. He was only five feet away from the bison, attempting to take a photo of it outside the Old Faithful Lodge, when the bison charged, goring him with its horns and tossing him into the air like a rag doll.

In June, a nineteen-year-old concession employee strolled too close to a bison after a late-night swim in the Firehole River, and the beast charged. Moments later, she too was airborne. Less than a week later, a sixty-eight-year-old woman was gored while on the Storm Point Trail overlooking Yellowstone Lake. And then, in July, a forty-three-year-old woman from Mississippi was posing for a picture in front of several bison—while holding her young daughter—when she heard the sound of hooves. They fled, but the bison caught them, and the woman was tossed. Luckily, her daughter was uninjured.

The victims in these attacks all survived, but the summer after I left Yellowstone, a baby bison wasn't so lucky. Thinking it was abandoned and cold, some well-meaning but misguided tourists placed the calf in their SUV and drove it to a ranger station. The rangers quickly released the young bison back into the wild, but since it had been handled by humans, the herd rejected it. When the calf wouldn't leave the roadway and started approaching cars, the park was forced to euthanize it.

As I struggled to keep the crowd of tourists away from the bison at Castle Geyser that afternoon, Drew, the security guard, wandered over. "Paramedics," he said, "always interfering with natural selection."

"Job security," I replied.

Drew hawked chewing tobacco into an empty Coke can. "You can't fix stupid."

"True," I said, telling Drew about a 9-1-1 call I'd run earlier that day at Gibbon Falls, thirty minutes north of Old Faithful.

Justin, a twenty-four-year-old motorcyclist from Billings, Montana, was having an allergic reaction, so he pulled over because his eyes were watering, and he couldn't see straight. When I arrived on-scene, I quickly determined he wasn't having a life-threatening anaphylactic reaction. When I asked to perform a physical exam, Justin was more concerned about his clothes than his health.

"Don't cut my riding pants!" he pleaded.

"I need to listen to your lung sounds and check for hives, swelling, or any trauma," I explained.

"Hell no," Justin protested, "I spent three hundred bucks on this riding outfit!"

Whether it was leather motorcycle pants, a skier's micro-polyester knit race outfit, or a scuba diver's wetsuit, years of working in EMS had taught me that, even when they're dying, patients cared more about their fashion.

Fortunately, Justin wasn't short of breath, his vital signs were normal, and he didn't have any throat or tongue swelling. However, he was traveling alone, and the symptoms hadn't resolved even after irrigating his eyes with normal saline. A bystander had already given him some Benadryl, and I recommended we take him to the Old Faithful Clinic or the hospital for additional evaluation.

"I'm concerned about your ability to safely drive your motorcycle," I explained. "Your eyes are watery, and you've taken Benadryl, which can make you drowsy."

Justin wasn't having it. "You're not gonna cut my riding pants or tell me what to do," he replied obstinately.

I informed Justin that riding a motorcycle through Yellowstone was dangerous. "We once had to call out six helicopters over the span of two days for motorcyclists who crashed after they drove to Yellowstone following the famous rally in Sturgis," I explained. "And that's not including the guy who slammed into the front of a pickup truck and died on-scene."

None of that mattered to Justin. "I ain't going."

He was alert and oriented so, by law, I couldn't make him go with us. If I did, I could actually be liable for false imprisonment or kidnapping according to US law. Instead, I had Justin sign the necessary refusal paperwork and told him to call us back at any time if his condition changed or worsened.

"Did he make it out alive?" Drew asked.

I told Drew I wasn't sure and then yelled at a tourist approaching the bison. "Move back! Twenty-five yards!"

The man scurried away as the alarm tones sounded on my pager. "Old Faithful EMS, respond to the West Entrance Road for a motorcycle accident."

"It couldn't be," I said.

Drew extended a betting hand. "Twenty-five bucks says it is!"

"Sorry!" I said, hurrying for the ambulance. "I don't have time to shake."

"You owe me!" Drew yelled.

I hopped in OF1 and gunned it, but before I made it to the Grand Loop Highway, dispatch cancelled me. The accident was near West Yellowstone, and Hebgen Basin Fire Department would take the call.

"OF1 standing down," I said over the radio. "Returning to Castle Geyser to prevent tourists from approaching bison."

Later that day, I learned that Drew had been right: it was Justin who'd been involved in the accident. He'd driven off the road and slammed into a tree. He survived the accident but was injured badly enough that Hebgen Basin requested a helicopter. Along with his injuries, Justin had an altered mental status which suggested a severe head injury or lack of oxygen to his brain—but he was sure of one thing.

"Don't cut my riding pants!"

IMMEDIATELY DANGEROUS TO LIFE AND HEALTH

IT DAWNED ON ME, out there in the woods and mountains and under the stars that seemed close enough to touch, that we were put here on this earth to help one another. My job as a paramedic—and as a person—was to never stop expanding the ways in which I could serve, protect, and save lives.

Like Cody, Sam, and many of the other rangers at Yellowstone, I wanted to become an all-hazards responder who could deploy anytime, anywhere, under any conditions to help someone and serve my country. Consequently, when Rachel, the district ranger who oversaw all of Old Faithful's law enforcement, fire, and EMS operations, called me into her office one day in August and offered me a chance to attend the National Park Service Structural Firefighting Academy—during which I'd learn to be a member of an engine company and fight blazes—I eagerly accepted.

The class was held at Glen Canyon National Recreation Area on the red-rock slot-canyon shores of Lake Powell. After weeks of online classes—which I completed after-hours and in between 9-1-1 calls at Old Faithful—I traveled to Glen Canyon with Zach for the practical portion of the class. The class was made up of personnel from all over the United States, who worked in every division of the NPS: law enforcement, interpretation, maintenance, field biology, and even graphic information system (GIS) mapping. There were even a few concession employees from Grand Canyon National Park.

Despite the differences in demographics, we all shared the goal of saving lives and protecting historic buildings, cultural resources, and valuable properties from fire. Along with responding to blazes, we'd learn vehicle extrication, forcible door entry, knots, how to raise ladders, and how to deal with hazardous material incidents.

On the first day, our class was separated into groups simulating a squad of firefighters who'd respond on an engine. Zach and I were assigned to team 3, along with a Thai American interpretative ranger from Zion named Dara, an LE ranger from Yosemite named Ernie, and a Mormon LE ranger from Bryce Canyon National Park.

"The name's Bryce," he said, extending his hand.

I gave him a funny look.

"Bryce," he said again. "And I also work in Bryce."

"Bryce from Bryce," I said, laughing. "Sounds like a great nickname to me!"

"Definitely," added Dara.

Dressed in heavy bunker gear—along with hoods, helmets, and self-contained breathing apparatus (SCBA)—while operating in desert temperatures that hovered around 100 degrees Fahrenheit, the members of team 3 struggled through rigorous training evolutions. We learned to launch an interior fire attack on a burning building, to follow a hose line in blackout conditions to rescue a downed firefighter, to follow the steps for calling a "Mayday, Mayday, Mayday!," to raise ladders, force doors, and cut holes in roofs with a chainsaw to perform vertical ventilation, and to extinguish a car fire and use the Jaws of Life to rescue a victim from a mangled vehicle.

As the course progressed, the evolutions became harder, longer, and more dangerous. We attacked a flaming "propane tree," fought vehicle fires, and used hydraulic tools like cutters, rams, and spreaders—the Jaws of Life—to cut up cars and rescue heavy mannequins that were trapped. The course culminated in a massive "live fire" scenario in which we'd have to enter a burning maze of shipping containers in blackout conditions to locate and extinguish a fire.

"You are about to enter an IDLH," announced Scott, one of our lead instructors. "That means the National Institute for Occupational Safety and Health has deemed it to be immediately dangerous to life and health."

Scott was a muscular guy with a drill-sergeant demeanor. He worked as a law-enforcement ranger at an East Coast park, firefighting being one of his collateral duties. Scott added that we'd been given the appropriate personal protective equipment, knowledge, skills, and training to be successful and safe during the evolution.

"Any questions?" he asked.

"No, sir," we said.

"Team 3," he said. "Are you a go for live fire?"

"Yes," we replied.

"I can't hear you," Scott said, raising his voice. "Are you a go for live fire?"

"We're a go for live fire," Dara, Zach, Bryce, and I said.

"ARE YOU A GO FOR LIVE FIRE?" Scott yelled, his neck veins bulging.

"TEAM 3 IS A GO FOR LIVE FIRE!" we hollered in unison, and then Scott told us to start the scenario and get it done.

We loved all our instructors, but especially Scott. He was super passionate, and, like a great coach, he was always encouraging us to do our best. We didn't mind his yelling either. Firefighting was a serious, and potentially deadly, business. We had to be ready.

In the burn box, the fire instructors lit a towering stack of wood pallets and waited for the steel shipping containers to get hot and fill up with blinding black smoke. Then they sent a training page over the radio: "Team 3, respond to a report of a structure fire at 100 Lake Shore Drive."

As we pulled up in the fire engine, I hopped off and connected our large-diameter hose line to a fire hydrant for a water supply. Bryce from Bryce assumed the role of incident commander and gave a scene size-up. "We have a single-story, fully-involved structure that is unvented at this time," he announced over the radio. "So we'll be performing an interior attack with door control."

The purpose of keeping the door as close to shut as possible and not breaking any windows was to control the flow path. The more air—and oxygen—we allowed into the structure, the bigger the fire would grow.

"Copy," replied Zach, pulling a two-hundred-foot section of hose line from the engine and hurrying it to the door.

Dara joined Zach at the door with a Halligan tool, pickaxe, and thermal imaging camera (TIC), which we'd use to find the seat of the fire and locate any victims.

After I finished with the hydrant, I hurried over to join Zach and Dara at the front door, and we donned our face masks, hoods, and helmets, went "on air," breathing from our SCBAs in deep, Darth Vader–like inhales and exhales, and assumed our place on the attack line. Zach was at the nozzle, Dara was behind him with the TIC and Halligan tool, and I was behind her with the pickaxe.

As we pried open the front door to the shipping container, turbulent black smoke billowed forth, and heat radiated like the container was an oven on the self-clean setting. Zach gave a few quick sprays into the building to cool the environment and then yelled, "Forward!" Dara and I grabbed the hose line and followed him, as Bryce from Bryce shut the door behind us until there was only a 1¾-inch opening, just wide enough for our hose to fit through.

Once inside, the intense heat immediately caused Zach, Dara, and me to drop to our hands and knees. It was coolest closest to the floor, but it was still scorching. We advanced, crawling forward with the hose line and fumbling around corners.

Zach unleashed a wall-ceiling-wall water pattern from the nozzle, yelling "Forward!"

He would move forward a few feet and then open up the nozzle, letting loose a hailstorm of water to cool the compartment, and then we'd plunge deeper into the structure. The smoke all around us was unburned fuel that could ignite at any moment, a deadly event known as a "flashover."

It grew even hotter as we advanced into the structure, squeezing around tight corners and crawling over toppled furniture in pitch-black smoke. I felt as if my liver and kidneys were roasting. I could see yellow and orange flames snaking through the smoke above and slithering down the walls in serpentine patterns. The spreading fire had a strange, intoxicating beauty. Part of me wanted to lie on my back and just watch the flames like passing clouds on a summer day. But everything about this IDLH environment—the heat, flames, and toxic gases—wanted me dead.

If Zach missed a hot spot or hidden pocket of flames, Dara or I would grab his shoulder and yell, "On the left!" or "Overhead!" and he'd quickly douse the area.

Suddenly we turned a corner, and the compartment got even hotter. Every survival instinct in me wanted to flee the area and crawl back to the door, but it wasn't about me any longer. I wasn't about to leave the other firefighters on the hose line. We were team 3, and this would be our finest hour.

Just then, Dara spotted the burning pallets in the corner of the room with the thermal imaging camera. "Back right corner!" she shouted, her voice sounding muffled through the face mask.

Zach turned and opened up the bale, letting loose with everything we had. As we hit the seat of the fire with 125 gallons of water per minute, the burning pallets sizzled and hissed like some prehistoric beast on its last breath, and the whole area cooled.

But our work wasn't done.

Performing a right-handed search along the wall, I found a window—wooden planks for this training scenario—and knocked it out with my pickaxe. Our goal now was to ventilate the structure and clear out all of the deadly black smoke.

"Incident command," Zach said over the radio, still struggling to catch his breath, "team 3 has fire knockdown," which meant the flames had been extinguished.

On the other side of the room, Dara punched out a window with her Halligan. As we called for ventilation, Bryce opened the front door to the burn box and activated a large positive pressure fan. It roared like a jet engine, and all of the smoke poured out of the structure in great gusts and mini tornadoes. Our visibility slowly returned and revealed an inch-deep soupy mix of soot, ash, and a few unburned wooden planks on the floor.

Scott waited for us as we emerged into the bright sunlight. "Strong work, team 3!" he yelled, helping us remove our SCBAs. "That's how you do it!"

Half an hour later, the burn box had been rehabbed, the instructors were lighting another pile of wood pallets, and Scott was pumping up another team of firefighters for the IDLH. "Team 4! Are you a go for live fire?"

Every student in my fire academy passed both the written and practical exam, and that evening we celebrated with sushi and sake at the Blue Buddha Lounge, just across the border in Page, Arizona. Before we left, Scott stopped by our table to congratulate us once again. "Just want to say it again, great job!"

We were all inspired by Scott's passion for firefighting and saving lives, and none of us would ever forget him. But there was a moment just before he left that made me worry. Scott said we could contact him anytime if we had a question about firefighting in the future. "Or anything else," he said, his eyes scanning the table to drive his point home. "You're my brothers and sisters now, and I'm here for you 24/7. This can be a tough profession."

We thanked Scott, but after he left, I wondered if he was talking about something beyond firefighting tools and tactics. Was there another side of being a first responder that concerned him?

I didn't have enough experience as an all-hazards responder to answer that night, but I would soon enough.

· · · · · · ·

Zach and I returned to Yellowstone, where we could now respond on Old Faithful's fire engine when the tones dropped. Most of the alarm activations were benign: steam from Park Service employees showering in the eight-plex and families cooking dinner on hot plates in their hotel rooms to avoid the high price of dining at the Old Faithful Inn. But when dispatch paged us out for a truck that rolled over, spilling five hundred gallons of yellow highway paint near Madison Junction one afternoon, I knew it was go time.

The truck driver was unharmed and self-extricated, but a thick, steady stream of yellow paint was coursing through the woods toward the Gibbon River. We'd all taken an oath to leave

Yellowstone "unimpaired for future generations," and now it was time to make good on that promise.

"We need to dam, dike, and divert this paint before it hits the river," Emily, the fire officer, yelled as we arrived on-scene.

Zach, Sam, Cody, and I grabbed shovels and rakes and began frantically moving dirt. We dug holes to catch the paint; crafted long, snake-like mounds to steer it; and assembled dams to stop it. But the yellow paint kept moving toward the river.

Due to the large volume, Emily quickly requested a professional hazardous material remediation team from Bozeman, but it'd take them at least two hours to respond.

"Faster," Emily yelled. "The paint is less than fifty yards from the river now."

The Gibbon flowed into the Madison River, and both were home to brown trout and trumpeter swans and provided an important water source for thousands of other animals, insects, and plants. In fact, the Madison River had been designated by the state of Montana as a Blue Ribbon Fishery, based upon its water quality, quantity, accessibility, and natural reproduction capacity for trout.

The paint was thirty yards away from the river's edge.

"Hurry!" Zach hollered, digging faster.

Just then, a cold drizzle began to fall. The rain mixed with the paint, reducing its viscosity, and causing it to flow faster. Zach, Sam, and I ramped up our efforts, but the paint kept moving.

"We're not going to be able to stop it!" I lamented.

"Tarps!" Emily suddenly yelled. "We'll cover the spill to prevent the paint from mixing with the rain!" Like all of Emily's ideas, it was audacious and improvised and just about the smartest plan I'd ever heard.

Twenty-five yards.

As Sam and I continued with our damming and diversion efforts, Emily and Zach quickly formed a grid with tent stakes and sticks and then placed sprawling red tarps on top, creating a roof above the spill. The falling rain made a rhythmic tapping sound on the tarps. Down the hill, Sam and I could immediately see Emily's solution working as the paint slowed its steady course toward the river.

Fifteen yards.

Zach and I had reached our "Alamo position," and it was time to give it everything we had. Sweating and exhausted, we built one final dam just before the river.

"Faster," I yelled, near collapse.

"I'm giving everything I got!" he replied.

Suddenly Emily and Sam called out to us. "Hey guys! You can stop now."

I looked up to see the spill had stopped moving. The river was saved.

"We did it!" I hollered.

Even better, the forest floor was comprised of a loose carpet of leaf litter, so when the hazardous cleanup crew arrived, they would likely be able to scoop it up, causing no lasting damage.

"Team 3 crushing it," Zach said, handing me a Gatorade.

"Always!" I replied, giving him a fist bump with my fire gloves.

We all felt proud to have protected the Gibbon River that afternoon, but as we drove back to Old Faithful, and the rain returned, there was something about the drops on the windshield and their tear-like trails down the glass that made me think of Scott again. "You are my brothers and sisters," he'd said.

In hindsight, I really wished we would've told him the same thing—that we were there for him too, 24/7. Would it have prevented the tragedy that transpired two years later? Maybe not. Probably not.

But maybe.

11

BE ON THE LOOKOUT

ALL UNITS BE ADVISED, I have eyes on the suspect," I announced over the radio.

Zach copied my traffic. "You found the BOLO?"

"Affirm."

"Location?"

"In the parking lot between the Old Faithful General Store and the gas station."

"Are you certain it's him?"

I peered into the binoculars again: the missing license plate, the silver 1988 Mazda 323 GTX, and—most importantly—the stolen items in the backseat. "It's him."

Zach told me to stay put and not to approach the suspect. "I'm en route from the ranger station."

People often went missing or committed crimes in national parks. Many criminals—like Charles Manson, who hid out in

Death Valley's Barker Ranch in 1968—also fled to national parks, seeking a safe haven. And when they did, LE rangers issued an alert known as a BOLO, short for "be on the lookout." BOLOs could be issued for a range of activities: driving under the influence, rape, theft, kidnapping, homicide, or simply going missing. A BOLO contained details about the suspect such as approximate age, race, height, weight, clothing, last known location, and direction of travel.

How did Hal Shipley from Twin Falls, Idaho, break the law that week in Yellowstone? A tourist had watched him fill the backseat of his car with rocks from the Upper Geyser Basin and reported it. It is a federal crime to remove any natural objects such as rocks, elk antlers, fossils, plants, or artifacts from a national park. Along with the goal of leaving the park "unimpaired for future generations," this law also recognizes that all organisms are interconnected and play an important part in the web of life. Hal's crime had been called in last night, but law enforcement rangers hadn't been able to locate him. Hence, the BOLO.

Along with the official BOLOs, there were also unofficial ones, designed to keep us alert, vigilant, and at times entertained. For example, when violent motorcycle gangs such as Hells Angels or the Mongols roared through the park, there was an unofficial BOLO for their whereabouts, direction of travel, and reports of anything suspicious. There was also a longstanding unofficial BOLO for the people who flocked to Yellowstone believing there was a treasure worth millions hidden somewhere within the park. According to lore, Forrest Fenn, a millionaire from Santa Fe, New Mexico, had buried the treasure somewhere in the Rockies and left clues in a poem he wrote, titled "The Thrill of the Chase."

Unfortunately for park rangers, these treasure seekers often arrived in the park terribly unprepared. They ventured forth into the wilderness at night without sleeping bags and attempted to descend the Grand Canyon of Yellowstone's steep cliff walls or cross raging rivers on cheap floats or self-made rafts. We kept an eye out for these scavengers because, based upon their ill preparation, it usually meant a search-and-rescue operation was about to ensue.

Some BOLOs were more lighthearted in tone. For example, when Sports Illustrated decided to shoot the Swimsuit Issue within the park, there was an unofficial BOLO among rangers—specifically male ones—to keep an eye out for Jessica Gomes, a bikini-clad supermodel posing at Grand Prismatic Spring and on the Old Faithful boardwalk.

Hannah and I had an unofficial BOLO for the Uinta ground squirrel that had moved into her trailer. Housing for seasonal employees of the Park Service ran the gamut from my cozy one-bedroom apartment to Hannah's dilapidated, moldy single-wide. She could tolerate the mice and the blue fungus crawling up her walls, but when the squirrel moved in, Hannah reached her limit. It all came to a head one afternoon when she fled from the squirrel into her bathroom and got stuck inside when the door broke. When I came to assist and attempted to open the door, the handle broke off in my hand.

"Sorry," I joked. "Guess I'll have to leave you there!"

Hannah reminded me that she saved us from coyotes that night at the upper geyser basin.

"Good point," I replied. "Time to use some of my new forcible entry firefighting skills."

Using some forcible entry skills I learned at the NPS Fire Academy, I managed to free Hannah, and a guy from facilities caught the squirrel a few days later.

One of the strangest BOLOs I encountered occurred in the weeks following a horrific car crash. On July 23, we responded to a head-on collision between a pickup truck and an SUV on the winding road between the Canyon and Norris Districts. We found multiple patients—some with life-threatening injuries—who were quickly transported to hospitals in Rexburg, Idaho, and Bozeman, Montana, by helicopter and ambulance. There was also a frightened dog in the backseat of the SUV in a travel crate. Jade was an adorable Australian Shepherd with blue eyes and a soft black-and-white coat that made me think of crumbled Oreo cookies. She'd survived the collision but then watched as her two injured owners—Laura Gillice and David Sowers from Denver—were evacuated from the scene emergently. As we approached the mangled SUV, Jade broke free of the crate, leapt from the truck, and disappeared into the woods. So an unofficial BOLO for an Australian Shepherd was issued.

When two weeks passed, we were certain Jade was dead. After all, she'd escaped into "America's Serengeti," populated with opportunistic predators like wolves, grizzly bears, and mountain lions.

While I didn't think I could help to find Jade, I could make a difference when it came to Hal Shipley and his stolen stones from the Upper Geyser Basin.

As Zach drove over to the general store from the ranger station that afternoon, he told me not to alert Hal of my presence, which could compromise my safety.

"Copy," I said, feeling more like 007 than my official call sign of 4-Oscar-20.

In hindsight, I couldn't have been more obvious: I was parked less than twenty-five yards from Hal's car; I had a pair of binoculars pressed to my eyes, and my ambulance announced Park Ranger in bold green letters.

But here's the thing: I was a paramedic seated in an ambulance, and no one ever suspects us. I was one of the good guys who saved your life in cardiac arrest or who gave you narcotics when you broke bones and sent you off to your warm, happy place.

"I'm not the cops," I'd often say to patients. "But do you have methamphetamine in this car with your daughter?"

I'm not the cops.

"Were you drinking alcohol before you hit that car?"

I'm not the cops.

"Did you hit your wife tonight?"

I'm not the cops.

"Your child has burns in a splash pattern. Did you dip her into hot bathwater?"

I wasn't a cop, but that didn't mean I wouldn't tell the police if people drove drunk, abused their spouse, hurt their children, or stole precious stones from fragile geyser basins.

Zach arrived a moment later and contacted with Hal Shipley. Hal was a disheveled man with tattered clothes who claimed to be a sovereign citizen.

"The United States government is illegitimate," Hal argued. "I don't have a social security number, driver's license, birth certificate, car registration, or a zip code, so you can't arrest me!"

Additional LE rangers arrived soon to provide backup. They removed the rocks, searched Hal's car, and took him into custody. He'd be transported up to the Mammoth District of Yellowstone where, if you can believe it, sat both a jail and a judge.

In the days following Hal's arrest, word of my catching the BOLO spread through the government area. OF1 was nicknamed the "undercover ambulance," and I started receiving text messages with the humorous #UA hashtag.

We had a good laugh about it, but when a legitimate BOLO was announced the morning of August 3 for Wade Tunstall, my heart dropped. For the last five years, Tunstall, a sixty-year-old man from Twin Falls, Idaho, had worked as a nurse at the Lake

District's medical clinic. According to the BOLO, Tunstall was last seen the day before at 11:00 am, and his fellow nurses had reported him missing when he didn't show up for work the following day.

We all gathered in the Old Faithful Ranger Station to brief on the case. I wanted desperately to conduct a search-and-rescue mission—meaning Tunstall was still alive—but I feared it might be what we called a body recovery. According to his coworkers, it was unlike Tunstall to disappear like that. Despite this, I mentally prepared myself to treat him as a paramedic, reviewing the protocols for trauma, hypothermia, crush injury, and dehydration.

Tragically, a team of rangers located Tunstall's body, with his "hiking boots protruding from a carnivore burial cache," a few hours later near a trail, just up the road from the Lake District's medical clinic. "The victim was found face down on his stomach with his left arm under his chest, and his left leg crossed over the calf of his right leg." An Interagency Board of Review, composed of state and federal personnel, would later conclude, "The body had been partially consumed and exhibited canine bite wounds and other injuries consistent with a bear attack. There were defensive (blocking type) bite wounds on Mr. Tunstall's right arm and both hands. Bruising associated with some wounds on the arms, hands, head, face, shoulders, and upper back indicated that Mr. Tunstall was alive at the time these wounds were inflicted. Tracks of an adult female grizzly bear and cub(s) were found next to the body and in day beds near the body."

I'd only met Tunstall once, briefly, when I stopped by the clinic to say hello. I didn't know him well, but he had a firm handshake and friendly demeanor, and he'd devoted as a nurse to helping people. In the end, what more do you need to know about someone?

Saddened, I decided to recommit to my job as a paramedic and honor Tunstall's legacy by protecting people in Yellowstone as best as I could.

"Rest easy, brother," I thought, "we'll take it from here."

· · · · · · ·

Fortunately, not all BOLOs ended with an arrest or body recovery.

Forty-two days after Laura Gillice and David Sowers were involved in the head-on collision, Laura was walking in the early-morning meadows of the Canyon District and heard the rustle of bushes. She turned and spotted a black-and-white blur racing toward her. The beast was gaunt and half wild, but Laura recognized the sweet bark and blue eyes. It was Jade, and she was coming home.

12

SINK OR SWIM

AND JUST LIKE THAT, I blinked, late September arrived, and my summer season at Yellowstone was coming to a close. I should've seen it coming by the Christmas-in-August celebration at the Old Faithful Inn on September 25, complete with carolers and a decorated tree; by the very clear terms of my summer appointment that stated, "Not to exceed 1039 hours"; by the concession employees' holding their survivor's party to celebrate the few that hadn't quit, been fired, or been arrested over the summer; and by the bugling elk and bison herds that were returning to the Old Faithful District, where the geysers and hot springs promised an element of warmth during the harsh winter months. I should've spotted the finish approaching, but when you don't want something to end, I guess you purposely try not to see the signs.

As I reflected upon my summer season, though, I couldn't have been happier. I'd spent the last five months living at the heart of one of the most magical places on the planet, working alongside some of the most dedicated and friendly people I'd ever met. I'd overcome my addiction to my cell phone, lessened my need to be constantly doing things, and felt more in touch with nature. In the space once occupied by busyness and technology, I was more open, receptive, connected, and alive.

I'd also grown tremendously as a paramedic. I was once a five-minute medic, skilled only at saving lives during the short transport time to a city hospital. But now I'd become proficient in treating patients in remote settings with limited resources and long transport times. However, two late-season calls at Yellowstone made me realize my process of learning wilderness medicine was just beginning.

One emergency occurred on the Mystic Falls Trail, high above Biscuit Basin, and involved us transporting a seventy-year-old woman with chest pain down the trail on a wheeled litter.

The second call occurred along the steep, boulderly banks of the Firehole River, eighty feet down from the road. Our patient that afternoon was a thirty-year-old attorney named Tina from Naples, Florida. She'd been rock hopping beside the river with her friends when she landed wrong and rolled her ankle. Since accessing Tina required us to travel down a steep, unmaintained trail with loose boulders, we couldn't just secure her to a backboard and carry her out. So Zach called for Yellowstone's rope rescue team. When it took the team around ninety minutes to travel to the incident site, I had my first taste of "prolonged field care," a term typically used when a provider has to treat a patient in the prehospital setting much longer than expected. As we waited for the rescue team, Sam and I treated Tina by splinting her ankle, starting an IV, administering pain medications, and checking her vital signs every thirty minutes. When the team arrived, I watched with awe as they set up a technical rescue system and extricated the woman to the ambulance using a wheeled litter, ropes, and pulleys.

As I pondered these two calls, I realized that a good number of my patient encounters at Yellowstone had occurred inside or quite close to buildings: hotel rooms, dorm rooms, parking lots, and geyser boardwalks. This was likely due to the fact that, for better or worse, 99 percent of Yellowstone's visitors typically stayed within a half mile of the road.

Despite the remoteness, I hadn't spent much time rescuing people on trails or learned a lot about search and rescue. There was an entire side of wilderness medicine I still hadn't experienced, and thus, I had a lot more to learn as a paramedic with the National Park Service.

Cody suggested I reach out to the EMS supervisor at Yosemite National Park. "They staff seasonal medics in the winter."

"That is, if he gets rehire status," joked Zach.

"Ha-ha," I replied, placing a new set of sheets on the gurney.

We were all at the Emergency Services Building, rehabbing OF1. I'd just returned from transporting a seventy-two-year-old man with shortness of breath and an irregular heartbeat from the Old Faithful Clinic to Rexburg, Idaho, via a rendezvous with Hebgen Basin Fire Department.

Suddenly, the alarm tones on our pagers sounded: *Old Faithful EMS, respond Alpha Priority to the Old Faithful Inn for a sixty-five-year-old woman with a diabetic complaint.*

"Alpha priority" meant dispatch had determined the call was nonurgent and requiring only basic life support.

"Who wants it?" asked Sam.

"I'll take it," I replied, hopping into the driver's seat. "And I'll call if I need any help."

"Thanks, buddy!" Cody said.

"Gotta get that rehire status!" I joked as I drove away.

Minutes later, I parked outside the Old Faithful Inn. Based on the dispatch notes, I was sure it would be a simple call: I'd take a set of vital signs, check the woman's blood sugar, and then, like many other nonemergencies, process the patient's refusal paperwork when the woman informed me she didn't want to leave her bus tour to go to the nearest hospital.

At least that's what I expected. But when I strolled into the hotel room, I found the bathroom floor covered in blood and Meryl Hinds from Birmingham, Alabama, slouched on the toilet in severe distress.

"Sink or swim," Cody had said four months earlier, when I asked what would happen if I ever ended up alone on the ambulance with a critical patient.

Meryl was actively dying in front of me, and I needed to do something fast.

But where to start?

Should I begin with her shortness of breath that had her struggling to speak, even in short one-word sentences? Or should I investigate her altered mental status that had her thinking she was back in Alabama? There was also the massive exsanguination—a slurry of blood and brown stool covering her, the wheelchair she used, and the bathroom floor. Or maybe I should start with the elephant in the room: why the hell did her husband, Petey, call 9-1-1 for a "mild diabetic complaint" when Meryl had all these other critical issues? It was the EMS equivalent of bringing a car with four flat tires, leaking fluid, and a dying engine to a mechanic and asking him to fix the cracked side mirror.

My first step in treating Meryl—a sickly woman with scars lining her arms and her right leg amputated below the knee—involved keying my radio and saying something along the lines of, "ShesDyingSendEveryoneAndLaunchAHelicopter!" in a rushed, panicky voice.

Petey, a tall, thin man with a long gray beard, stepped in close. "I think her blood sugar's a little off."

I didn't even respond. Politeness went by the wayside when you were alone with a critical patient. Instead, I grabbed a towel off the rack and handed it to Meryl. The toilet was filled with bloody stool, so it was clear she had had a massive GI bleed.

"Place this towel between your legs and apply pressure to stop the bleeding," I commanded from the bathroom doorway.

Next, I gave her supplemental oxygen to help with her respiratory distress, and I was just about to storm into the bathroom—bloody boots and uniform be damned—to get a set of vital signs and start an IV when Petey informed me Meryl had a history of diabetes, cirrhosis (or scarring) of the liver, chronic obstructive pulmonary disease, MRSA, and Hepatitis C.

The scene came to a screeching halt. MRSA (methicillin-resistant Staphylococcus aureus) is a highly contagious, antibiotic resistant—and potentially deadly—staph infection that's spread through skin-to-skin contact. Hepatitis C is a viral infection that causes liver failure and is spread through infected blood.

I keyed my radio and gave the responding units another order. "Wear everything!" By that, I meant the personal protective equipment that would keep us all safe.

While I wasn't about to get bloody, I could still treat Meryl and help save her life. She had a weak pulse at her wrist, and when I placed a pulse oximeter on her finger, I found her heart rate elevated.

She's in compensated shock, I thought. *Her fast pulse is desperately trying to make up for the loss of blood volume.* I knew she could further deteriorate at any moment and go into cardiac arrest.

"Hang in there, ma'am," I said. "My team is coming to help you."

Outside, I heard the rising and falling whine of sirens in the distance, growing louder, ripping open the silent Old Faithful night.

Sam, Zach, and Cody soon arrived, wheeling in the gurney and carrying kits of personal protective gear for us. On went the yellow isolation gowns, on went the clear chemical impact goggles, the blue ear-loop face masks and exam gloves.

"Helicopter is inbound with a fifteen-minute ETA," said dispatch.

We quickly loaded Meryl onto the gurney, covered her with a blanket, and wheeled her through the historic hallways of the Old Faithful Inn, passing dozens of tourists. They were all dressed mountain casual, strolling to their rooms with bellies full of bison burgers and osso buco. We looked like the government operatives in hazmat suits from the escape scene in E.T., racing down the hall, all "Nothing to see here, folks!"

Once we arrived at the ambulance, we quickly loaded Meryl and gunned it toward the Old Faithful Ranger Station. En route, we checked her vital signs, obtained a 12-lead EKG to look at her heart rhythm, and gave her a breathing treatment with the drug albuterol, to help with her shortness of breath and wheezes.

A typical blood pressure is around 120/80, and we found Meryl's dangerously low at 75/55. We needed to start an IV immediately and administer saline, but she had track marks lining her arms from years of drug abuse, so I couldn't find a vein. Fortunately, when the flight crew arrived a few minutes later, they placed an IV and started giving Meryl fluid to raise her blood pressure.

A storm had rolled in by then, and great gusts of wind and rain pummeled the Old Faithful Ranger Station.

"Feel better, Meryl," I said as I closed the helicopter door.

The bird lifted from the LZ soon after, straining against the wind, only to land a few seconds later.

"Can't fly in this weather," said the pilot, hopping out and yelling above the gale.

I was already planning for this kind of contingency.

"We can drive to West Yellowstone and request a fixed-wing airplane," I said without a second thought.

"Perfect," Sam replied. "I'll drive.

We loaded Meryl into the back of the ambulance, the flight paramedic and nurse jumped in with me, and off we roared down the Grand Loop Highway, dodging bison and elk along the way.

En route, Meryl began nodding off and becoming less responsive. Would she stop breathing? Go into cardiac arrest?

"Her pupils are pinpoint," I declared, shining a penlight. "She might have overdosed on narcotics too!"

"I'll grab the Narcan to reverse it," declared the flight nurse, reaching for the thin, pink medication box that had saved so many lives over the years.

The fixed-wing was able to land in West Yellowstone that night, and we flew Meryl out. Miraculously, she'd make it to the hospital alive. In Idaho Falls the doctors would diagnose her with a massive GI bleed, shock, a COPD exacerbation, narcotic overdose, and—thanks, Petey—a "diabetic complaint."

Meryl's blood sugar was mildly elevated.

· · · · · · ·

I wasn't sure if it was the way I handled the call with Meryl or my overall performance over the summer, but Rachel called me into her district ranger office the following week and handed me my employee evaluation. "Great work," she said. "And congrats, you have rehire status!"

I was thrilled with the achievement, but I knew I had a lot more to learn about wilderness medicine and becoming an all-hazards responder to best serve my community.

Hannah left that week to spend the winter in Joshua Tree National Park in California, where she'd give ranger-led programs on the flora and fauna of the desert and the unique night sky, devoid of light pollution and perfect for watching stars.

"I'll carry your things to your car," I told her, grabbing a heavy box full of field guides, hiking books, and a book by her favorite poet, Mary Oliver.

Hannah's departure day had arrived, and I was about to learn a tough lesson about seasonal employment with the NPS: relationships can be time-stamped.

Hannah said she had a great summer getting to know me, but she didn't think we'd see much of each other in the future. "You want to move back to Southern California and work for a fire department in Los Angeles," she began. "I'm not a huge fan of cities and crowds and am considering graduate school."

I couldn't argue.

Hannah gave me a hug. "Just don't forget to follow your heart."

"What do you mean?" I asked, pulling away.

"You seem really happy here," she said. "This is your tribe. Your roots are in the mountains."

I hugged her again and then waved as she drove off, feeling free in a weird kind of way.

My cell phone rang a few days later. It was the EMS supervisor at Yosemite. "We'd like to hire you as a paramedic for the winter. Interested?"

Like Yellowstone, millions of tourists flock to Yosemite every year, and the park had a high EMS call volume, including hundreds of search-and-rescue missions.

"Yes, I'd love to!" I replied.

I bid farewell to my Old Faithful friends—Sam, Cody, Emily and Zach, the volunteers, clinic staff, and the rest of my campfire community—and then packed my bags and pointed my car toward the Range of Light: the Sierra Nevada.

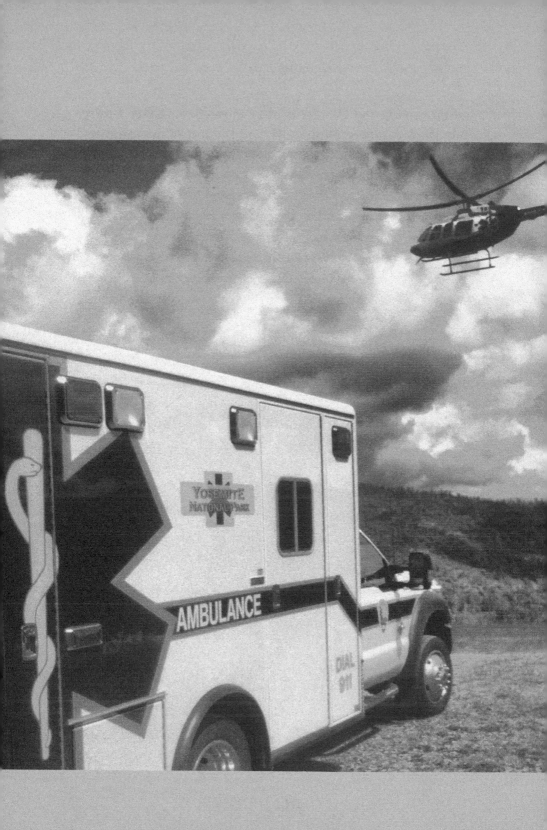

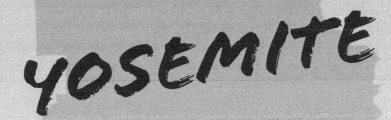

PART II

YOSEMITE

37.7456° N, 119.5936° W

It is by far the grandest of all the special temples of Nature I was ever permitted to enter.

—John Muir

13

THE OTHER "Y" PARK

FIRST PROTECTED IN 1864 and later expanded and designated as a national park in 1890, Yosemite boasts over 747,000 acres of dense forests, towering granite cliffs, tumbling waterfalls, and ancient sequoia groves.

Millions of tourists visit both Yellowstone and Yosemite annually, but I was told to expect a more active visitor in Yosemite: hikers ascending the cables leading to Half Dome's steep summit, illegal BASE jumpers launching themselves off cliffs in wingsuits, slack liners testing their balance—and safety harnesses—high above Yosemite Falls, rock climbers, and other intrepid souls, like those who soared high above the valley floor on a rope swing, known as the Porch Swing, attached to the southeast wall of the three-thousand-foot iconic rock face of El Capitan.

"Yosemite is a trauma park," the EMS supervisor for Yosemite, Sarah Pardee, had told me during our phone interview. "You'll see it all here."

Like Yellowstone, Yosemite's scenic wonders seemed matched only by the ways in which the park could extinguish you. For example, 162,000 tons of rock suddenly let loose on the Happy Isles Trail in 1996, wounding eleven people and killing one. In 2011, three hikers were swept over Vernal Falls and plunged 317 feet to their death. In 2012, two brothers, aged six and ten, fell into the swift Merced River during a family trip, both perishing. A California man climbed Matthes Crest alone in 2014 to celebrate proposing to his girlfriend hours earlier, only to fall three hundred feet to his death. On another grim occasion, an oak tree fell and struck the tent of two campers, killing them.

Yosemite didn't have grizzlies or sharp-horned bison who targeted selfie-taking tourists, but black bears and mountain lions populated the park, and heck, even the mice were dangerous. A hantavirus outbreak, spread by the urine, feces, and saliva of mice, infected ten people in 2012, killing three. Along with the outdoor dangers, there was also an urban element in Yosemite. Back in 1970 chaos broke out when hundreds of hippies wouldn't leave Stoneman Meadows, and park rangers were forced to use nightsticks, ropes, and Mace to control the unruly, drunken crowd. More recently, norovirus outbreaks have sickened hundreds, and problems have arisen with gang members from the Central Valley who flock to the park to deal drugs, flee arrest warrants, and tag boulders with graffiti.

My arrival in the other Y park started promisingly enough. As I drove into the park via the west entrance and emerged from the cool mosquito shadows of Wawona Tunnel, the Yosemite Valley appeared before me in all of its splendor: a magnificent U-shaped panorama of dense forests, plunging cascades, and the granite massifs of Half Dome, El Capitan, and Clouds Rest. However, from that majestic, sun-soaked promontory, Highway 41 dipped back into the woods, storm clouds massed overhead, and shadows splashed across the road as I descended toward the valley. I felt as if I were descending into the belly of some mythological beast. By the time I reached the valley floor, a light drizzle dotted my windshield, and my wipers made rhythmic whooshes across the glass. Gazing up at the fortress-like granite walls, I had a palpable sense of nature's danger, indifference, and death.

I followed Southside Drive as it wound through the valley, snaking alongside the tumbling Merced River and passing a tiny chapel before taking a right toward the medical clinic.

At Yosemite, I wouldn't have the luxury of my own one-bedroom apartment. Instead, I'd reside in a five-bedroom dorm situated across the parking lot from the medical clinic. Sarah had described "Casa de Medicos" as a legendary abode that frequently hosted campfires, potlucks, and parties. However, when I arrived that November afternoon, I found the place strangely empty.

"Hello," I called out, knocking. "Anyone here?"

Silence.

The side door was open, so I followed a narrow hallway past four bedrooms—each one bursting with outdoor gear like climbing ropes, helmets, bouldering crash pads, and carabiners—into a spacious kitchen and living room area complete with a ping-pong table, its green surface dotted with red Solo cups. I spotted an unclaimed room, began unpacking my car, and over the course of that rainy afternoon, met my four roommates.

Noah Hills, twenty-six, was a baby-faced, brown-eyed surfer and climber from Oxnard, California, with a slight beach bum vibe. He'd started in Yosemite as a volunteer with Yosemite Search and Rescue (YOSAR), spending the summer living in one of the tent cabins at legendary Camp 4. In 2003, Camp 4 was placed on the National Register of Historic Places because of its influence on the modern rock-climbing era, thanks to legendary climbers like Warren Harding, Royal Robbins, and Yvon Chouinard (the founder of Patagonia), who launched epic first ascents up Yosemite's towering granite walls in the 1950s and '60s. After that, Noah had attended paramedic school in Ventura and was now back at Yosemite. His plan was to spend a few years in the valley practicing emergency medicine and climbing before returning to school to become a physician's assistant.

Upon first meeting Ben Ford—a tall, laid-back guy from the Bay Area with a perpetual five o'clock shadow—I witnessed him asking if he could have some of Noah's hummus and then watched as he devoured the entire family-sized container in seconds. I quickly learned that Ben was like a human garbage disposal and bummed all his meals or just took scraps from whatever dish someone else couldn't finish. He was the ultimate mooch, but so cool and friendly that none of us ever minded. Ben had an endearingly unkempt quality—a button undone here, a zipper there—and had a hard time waking up for calls at night. When the alarm tones sounded, you'd hear him in his room like a gathering storm, struggling to get dressed, crashing into furniture, and then he'd appear moments later, saying, "Let's go. I'm ready!" while no doubt missing some important item like a shoe or his duty shirt.

"Hey," said Joel Hawk, my third roommate, hurrying past.

"Nice to meet y—," I said, watching him go.

Joel was a high-strung guy from Louisiana. He'd originally worked in a busy urban EMS system and came to the park seeking a remedy from burnout.

"We're very similar," I said, "only instead of New Orleans, I'm hoping to work in Los Angeles after a brief stint in the national parks."

"Are you kidding me?" Joel asked. "I'm never going back to the city!"

Joel said he loved remote medicine and working for the NPS. His plan was to spend a few years working as a paramedic and then become a law enforcement ranger.

"Welcome to Yosemite," said my fourth housemate, Luke Cohen, a handsome LE ranger from Colorado. Ever meet someone who excelled at everything, never broke a sweat, and was also good-looking? That was Luke. Like some James Bond of firefighting and EMS, he was well-educated, astute, charming, debonair, and always had a beautiful girl on his arm. Plus, no matter what the emergency, he could save your life anytime or anywhere. You almost wanted to hate him for it, but Luke was so friendly and humble that you couldn't.

And on most nights, we also had a fifth roommate who wasn't any specific person. Rather, it was whoever was crashing on the couch in our living room on that particular night. Some nights it was a "SAR siter," a search-and-rescue volunteer who lived in the tent cabins at the SAR site, Camp 4, and sought a shower and tasty meal. Sometimes our fifth roommate was a climbing bum from Camp 4, also in search of a hot shower and a home-cooked meal. Other nights during my time at Yosemite, my fifth roomie was one of Noah's or Luke's climbing buddies; or even, at times, a complete stranger—a friend of a friend of a friend—who didn't have a place to sleep because the campgrounds were all sold out.

That night, our fifth roommate was Lance Scott, a bespectacled guy in his midtwenties from Oregon with wild hair and Silicon Valley smarts who also, evidently, climbed like a spider monkey. Lance had spent the summer and the first part of fall working as a YOSAR volunteer at Tuolumne Meadows, and now he was off to Denver to attend paramedic school. His goal was to get his medic certification and return to the NPS to work as a climbing ranger at a park like North Cascades, Yosemite, Rainier, or Rocky Mountain.

That evening, as Joel and Noah whipped up a chicken stir-fry—and Ben waited in the wings for them to say "when"—I heard more about the types of EMS calls I could expect in Yosemite.

"We get a ton of SARs," Noah explained, referencing search and rescues.

"And most begin with the callers saying they're off-trail, lost, don't have a flashlight, and have a cell phone that's dying," added Joel, shaking his head with frustration.

As I ate stir-fry and later joined in a spirited game of ping-pong, my new roommates seemed friendly enough, but I had a sense they were sizing me up. Was I just insecure? Or would life be different at the epicenter of the climbing world, a hypercompetitive rock garden of first ascents and free solos?

I'd heard from other LE rangers that working in Yosemite was different than other busy districts in the National Park Service, like Old Faithful or the South Rim of the Grand Canyon. While relations had improved in recent years, there was a long history of overly stern law enforcement rangers clashing with laid-back rock climbers that made "the valley shift," the unofficial term rangers used to describe the Visitor and Resource Protection Division, seem at times more NYPD than NPS. I'd been immediately accepted into the tribe at Yellowstone, but I could tell I'd have to earn my way into Yosemite's elite rescue community. So when Sarah, my EMS supervisor, asked for a volunteer the following day, I quickly raised my hand.

"Great!" she said. "We're going to need you to don full personal protective gear for an Ebola drill."

The goal of the training scenario that afternoon was to run a mock emergency in which a patient showed up at the Yosemite Medical Clinic with the telltale signs and symptoms of Ebola, a highly contagious disease spread through direct contact with blood or other bodily fluids. In the training scenario, we'd have to take the necessary isolation precautions before treating and transporting the patient to Mercy Ambulance at El Portal, a small town near the Arch Rock entrance to the park. As had been the case at Yellowstone, the closest hospital and trauma centers were hours away, so we'd often hand off a patient via a rendezvous with another service like Mercy Ambulance or Sierra Ambulance. This allowed us to return to the park to provide coverage.

The training 9-1-1 page went out: "Ambulance 3, please respond to the medical clinic for a patient with flu-like symptoms who's recently traveled to Africa."

I was the lead patient care provider, so I threw on the personal protective gear: a white fluid-resistant suit, face mask, goggles, hood, heavy boot and shoe covers, and then sealed and reinforced every seam with duct tape.

"How you doing in there?" Noah asked.

"What?" I yelled.

"HOW YOU DOING IN THERE?"

"GOOD!" I replied, immediately drenched in sweat.

As we loaded the mock patient—Ben, who had perpetual bed head—into the ambulance and started driving the winding road toward El Portal, nausea set in. I broke out in a cold sweat and felt the color draining from my face.

"YOU OK?" Noah yelled.

He was also dressed in full PPE, although he didn't seem to be suffering the motion sickness afflicting me.

"PERFECT!" I replied, swallowing my rising stomach acids.

Luckily, I didn't puke on the drive to El Portal, but the moment we handed the patient over to the crew from Mercy Ambulance, I tore off my protective gear and sat on the curb, struggling to catch my breath.

"Have some water," Sarah instructed me. "You look a little green."

"Don't worry," Ben said. "Our medical director has authorized us to take Zofran every time we feel sick."

Since I'd essentially ripped off my suit, Sarah told me I'd lost points on the portion of the training that covered correct removal of the PPE. As I looked around at Noah, Luke, Joel, and Ben, I could see doubt in their eyes, and I wondered if I'd made a horrible mistake in coming to Yosemite. Would I ever fit in if I didn't rock climb? Could I work as a paramedic if I got car sick in the back of the ambulance?

Frustrated, I questioned the relevance of the training that day. "What are the odds of someone with Ebola ever showing up in Yosemite Valley?"

Joel laughed. "Actually, the odds are pretty good."

As luck would have it, the physician's assistant who lived with his family directly behind Casa de Medicos was—at that very hour—working at an Ebola treatment unit in Monrovia, Liberia, and he'd be returning to the park the following week.

I imagined the contagion sweeping through the valley, creating hysterical fear and paranoia. The fact that I'd be living in an isolated community next to a guy who'd just returned from Liberia and whose children—those little vectors of transmission—loved to visit their cool "uncles" at Casa de Medicos, was just another reason accepting this job at Yosemite might've been a very bad decision.

But I wouldn't give up that easy.

If there was anything I'd learned working as a paramedic, it was that the moment you feel like running away is when you should commit to trying harder. So when a call came in shortly thereafter that a climber had fallen on El Capitan, I said a quick prayer and raced for the ambulance. As in Yellowstone, I had to complete a weeklong field training before I was able to operate on my own in the back of the ambulance. That day, Joel, with his anxious, twitching energy, was working on the ambulance with me, and his stern paramilitary manner reminded me of my preceptors in Los Angeles during paramedic school.

I decided my comeback would begin right then, with the rock climber we found seated in the grass.

"What hurts?" I asked Bill, a twenty-six-year-old hippie with ropey dreadlocks from North Conway, New Hampshire.

"My ankle," he replied pointing.

Bill's ankle and lower leg had been secured in a makeshift splint: a sleeping pad, secured with silver tape.

"Duct it or fuck it," his buddy said with a stoner laugh. "It was all we had."

I instructed Joel to obtain Bill's vital signs, and I questioned him about the fall. He said he was climbing the twenty-fifth pitch of El Capitan and fell approximately thirty feet, slamming his left ankle on a ledge. After the accident, Bill's climbing partner splinted his leg, and then they rappelled down to El Capitan Meadow and called 9-1-1.

"Did you lose consciousness when you fell?" I asked, performing a rapid trauma exam.

"Nah, bro."

"Does anything else hurt?"

Bill said his lower back and chest hurt a bit, but he guessed it was probably due to his climbing harness.

"Vital signs within normal limits," Joel announced, removing the blood pressure cuff from Bill's arm.

"Copy," I replied, smiling to myself. This was just the softball 9-1-1 call I needed to get back on track.

But when I proposed my treatment plan to Bill, it took an odd turn: he refused everything.

"I'd like to expose your ankle to check your circulation, motor and sensory."

"It's already splinted," Bill replied. "Just leave it."

"Based on the height of the fall and your back pain," I said, "I'd like to place you in a full-body vacuum splint."

"Not necessary, but thanks."

I asked if I could start an IV.

"Nah."

"You don't want pain medication?"

"I'm good."

Suddenly, the call that I thought would turn everything around became simply basic life support. Flabbergasted, I asked Bill why he'd dialed 9-1-1 if he didn't want us to help him.

"I need a lift to the hospital," he said with a chuckle. "No car, bro!"

We loaded Bill into the back of the ambulance and drove to the south entrance, the Wawona Tunnel, where we met an EMS team from Sierra Ambulance. En route, my car sickness returned, and I had to pop a Zofran and crack a window to avoid vomiting.

Since I hadn't performed any interventions, Joel said this call wouldn't count toward my credentialing process, but my bigger concern was that I was getting car sick every time I rode in the back of the ambulance. And I knew I would never finish my field training, or be able to work as a paramedic in Yosemite, if I was always more ill than my patients.

As the shift ended, Noah told me not to worry. He said the critical calls would come, and the following day a call proved him right. When a concession employee with a history of seizures was found wandering around his building in the Curry Village dazed and with blood trickling out of his right ear, Noah and I responded with lights and sirens.

Leroy was a fifty-four-year-old bald man with twitchy eyes and long, unkempt eyebrows. He was sitting anxiously on his bed.

"What happened?" Leroy asked.

"It sounds like you had a seizure," I replied.

Leroy was able to answer basic questions—time, date, and location—but there was a large circle of dried blood on his carpet that appeared to have leaked from his right ear canal. Had Leroy seized, causing him to fall and hit his head? Or had he passed out, hit his head, and *then* started seizing due to a traumatic brain injury? Was the dried blood on the carpet from the tympanic membrane of his eardrum? Or was it a sign of a life-threatening basilar skull fracture? There was only one answer as to what to do next.

"Launch a helicopter," I said to Noah and Ben.

So much of being a good patient care provider comes down to experience. If you've seen an illness or injury once, you can more easily spot it a second time. At Yellowstone, I'd run a call for an eight-year-old boy who fell off the Old Faithful boardwalk, hit his head, and also had blood seeping out of his ear.

Anne, the PA at the clinic, had said there was no way to determine if it was a skull fracture or ruptured eardrum in the prehospital setting, so we'd ended up flying the boy to Idaho Falls. (That is, once the angry bull bison moved off the landing zone at Old Faithful, and we could land the chopper.)

I quickly told Noah and Ben this story and reasserted my transport plan, "Fly him."

"Negative on the air ambulance," Ben said. "It can't land in the valley at night due to the high rock walls."

"Copy," I replied. "Let's transport him to El Portal for a rendezvous with Mercy Ambulance."

En route, Ben and I placed an IV, checked Leroy's heart rhythm, and ensured he didn't get low on oxygen or drop his blood pressure. An instance of either condition—hypoxia or hypotension—would greatly increase his chance of dying. As we raced toward El Portal, Leroy kept repeating what he was saying—known as *perseverating*—which signaled he might have a significant brain injury.

"It feels like someone is sticking a needle in my ear," Leroy said.

"I'm sorry, sir," I said, placing a hand on his shoulder. "We're doing the best we can."

"It feels like someone is sticking a needle in my ear."

"You'll be at the hospital shortly," I said, "and they can give you something for the pain."

"It feels like someone is sticking a needle in my ear."

As we raced toward our rendezvous spot, all my energy and attention were focused on Leroy. Nothing existed in the world except comforting him and monitoring his vital signs. When we arrived at El Portal, we quickly transferred him to the paramedics with Mercy Ambulance, and they gunned it for John C. Fremont Hospital, a tiny medical facility in the town of Mariposa. There, doctors would perform a CT scan of Leroy's head and, if necessary, request a helicopter.

Leroy was diagnosed with a basilar skull fracture and a small brain bleed and ended up spending a few weeks in the hospital. Driving back into the valley that night, it dawned on me that I hadn't gotten carsick. Focusing all my energy and attention on my patient proved to be a better antidote to nausea than Zofran.

Maybe I can work in Yosemite! I thought.

· · · · · · ·

A few shifts later, I was officially cleared and allowed to operate on my own in the back of the ambulance. I was excited, though I still sensed it would take longer for me to actually break into the inner valley shift circle here, especially with Joel. We hadn't exactly hit it off as friends, probably because we'd both worked in busy urban

EMS systems and were too alike, but I resolved to keep trying to make a connection.

One evening in late November, I met Brad Miller, the physician's assistant at the clinic. He had recently returned from his deployment with the World Health Organization, treating Ebola patients in Liberia and was now back in the village on a mandatory quarantine period. Standing a few feet apart, we exchanged pleasantries, and I could tell I'd enjoy working with him and would learn a lot.

But he didn't shake my hand, and I didn't reach out to shake his.

14

LUG-NUT RULE

DURING OUR TRAUMA LECTURES at paramedic school, we'd studied the classical branch of mechanics known as kinematics, which took a detailed look at the movement and collision of objects and bodies. We memorized Sir Isaac Newton's first law of motion—*Every object will remain at rest or in uniform motion in a straight line unless compelled to change its state by the action of an external force*—and committed the formula for kinetic energy to memory. We learned there were three collisions in every car accident—the vehicle with the object, the driver with the vehicle, and the internal organs of the occupant as they sheared and collided. And, lastly, we watched gruesome online videos that showed, in horrific display, that the shorter the stopping distance, the more force from the impact was transferred to the occupant, resulting in major trauma.

Like the Park Service's investigative unit, NPS's version of CSI, we were taught to analyze accident scenes, asking: *Was there air bag deployment? Was the windshield splintered in a spiderweb-like shape, suggesting the driver's head hit the glass? Did the driver go up and over the steering wheel? Or down and under, into the wheel well?*

The goal of this detailed analysis was to identify the mechanism of injury and forces involved, so we could quickly identify critical patients. It was important knowledge—but Drew, the security guard at Yellowstone, had once offered a far simpler formula: "Just follow the lug-nut rule," he told me as we'd stood together near the Old Faithful Lodge one afternoon, informing tourists that no, their children couldn't ride the bison. "He who has the most lug nuts wins. It's true in NASCAR and in trauma."

I didn't quite understand.

"Your more critical patients will always be found in the vehicle with less lug nuts."

I was skeptical that Drew's lug-nut rule could usurp Sir Isaac Newton—the "father of modern science"—but it proved correct later that summer when a tiny Honda veered across the yellow median and collided head-on with a Chrysler Town & Country minivan. The lug-nut rule was right on when a Suburban rear-ended a small Kia Rio that braked suddenly at the Old Faithful roundabout and when a motorcyclist slammed into a Ford pickup near Lewis Lake, killing the biker instantly.

Every time I rolled up to one of these incidents, I thought of Drew's theory and immediately went to the smaller vehicle with fewer lug nuts, which was where I almost always found the most critical patients.

However, like all formulas, Drew's theory had its exceptions, especially in the context of a national park where moving vehicles often collided with other objects containing no lug nuts at all. For example, Drew's theory didn't hold when we responded to a motorcyclist who'd broadsided a bison one dark night on the Grand Loop Highway in Yellowstone or when a Toyota Tacoma skidded on black ice and slammed into a large ponderosa pine in Yosemite.

Twenty minutes earlier, Brendon Evans and his girlfriend, Melissa, had been driving into the valley when they hit a patch of black ice and took an unplanned tour of Yosemite's dense woods. Their truck hit the tree with such speed—and at such an angle— that the steering wheel bent toward Melissa, and the driver's side airbag deployed in her direction. Encased by air bags in all directions, her experience of the crash was sudden but soft, more bounce house than bad car accident. Brendon's experience was all twisted metal and solid wood with fifty-five miles per hour of impact.

Brendon was visiting Yosemite from Reno, Nevada, where he wore Brooks Brothers suits and worked as a criminal defense attorney. But now, as I approached his mangled truck that cold November morning, he was a bloody mess of a man, pinned in the driver's seat, frothing at the mouth, and yelling incoherently. His 2012 Toyota Tacoma was wrapped around the deep-rooted ponderosa. Despite its lack of lug nuts, the tree had clearly won this battle.

"Hang tight," I said through the driver's side window. "My team is going to get you out."

Brendon continued thrashing wildly and screaming.

In Hollywood, people reacted nobly to trauma. Despite being shot or stabbed, they always seemed able to crack a half smile and summon a short breath to say, "Go on without me" or "I love you." However, in real life a critical trauma call was always a messy and chaotic affair during which, rather than giving thanks for our EMS efforts, patients were often combative.

As firefighters worked to free Brendon with the Jaws of Life, I checked in with Melissa. After the accident, she had been able to self-extricate and dial 9-1-1.

"Sure you're not injured?" I asked.

Melissa told me she was fine. "But I'm worried about him," she said. Staring down at her hands, she added, "I think he was going to propose to me tonight."

"Don't worry, ma'am," I said. "We're doing everything we can."

Somewhere deep in the crushed wreck, Brendon was still yelling and struggling. Through the dented metal, I could see he had a large laceration on the right side of his head, plus what appeared to be two broken femurs and a busted wrist, dangling limply. Despite those gruesome injuries, I was most concerned with his altered mental status and combativeness. He likely had a significant head injury, and his agitation was increasing the swelling in his brain. That swelling would soon decrease blood flow and the delivery of oxygen, causing him to die.

I wanted to administer Versed, a sedative, to calm him, but I knew the medication could just as easily knock out his respiratory drive and the fight-or-flight response that was keeping him alive by elevating his heart rate and maintaining his blood pressure. If I gave him Versed while he was still trapped, and his vital signs tanked, I couldn't revive him.

As the firefighters continued working to extricate Brendon, using the Jaws of Life to peel away layers of the car like some grotesque, metallic onion, I held off giving the medication.

Time passed. Too many minutes. Brendon was growing more agitated, howling primordially like a caged animal, and I feared he would lose a pulse at any moment.

Desperate, I called dispatch to request a medevac, but none were available. It seemed like a cruel joke; the skies above Yosemite Valley were clear, but evidently, the helicopter launch site in the Central Valley was socked in with pea-soup fog.

"No life flights today," I said to Joel. "Gotta drive this one toward Fresno once we extricate him."

The trauma center in Fresno was over two and a half hours away.

"Copy," he replied. "Let's get the ambulance ready."

While the firefighters continued working, Joel and I hopped into the ambulance to crank the heat and prep IV supplies, bags of saline, and spinal immobilization equipment.

We'd been on-scene for over twenty minutes, and I knew our tactics needed to change. We'd made little progress in extricating Brendon. *The definition of insanity is doing the same thing over and over and expecting a different result.* Suddenly, I spotted the winch cable on the front of the light rescue apparatus parked nearby and remembered Emily's audacious—and ultimately, life-saving—decision to use it to haul our obese patient up the steep hillside in Yellowstone. I noticed a tow hitch on the rear of the Toyota Tacoma. *What if instead of trying to move Brandon from the truck, we freed the vehicle from the tree?*

Joel must've been thinking the same thing because he suddenly blurted out, "The winch cable and tow hitch!"

As we shared our idea with the firefighters, they immediately agreed, and a sense of momentum returned to the scene. We quickly attached the cable to the tow hitch, and moments later the truck was freed from the tree.

The extrication team of firefighters located a small crack, or "pinch point," amid the wrinkled metal and inserted the mighty blades of a hydraulic tool to pop the driver's side door off.

Brendon was still combative, so I administered an intramuscular injection of Versed into his right deltoid, more confident now that he was free of the vehicle. As he calmed, we quickly applied a cervical collar and then moved him onto a backboard and into the ambulance. En route, Joel and I checked Brendon's vitals, placed two IVs, administered 4mg of Zofran, splinted his broken legs and wrist, gave him a headband of gauze to stop the bleeding from the laceration on his head, and checked his heart rhythm. His condition stayed the same throughout the transport, and we met paramedics from Sierra Ambulance at the Wawona General Store. They would race him toward Fresno and, if possible, land a helicopter along the way.

Once we passed him over to Sierra, Joel and I rehabbed the ambulance. The past few days had been a little rough, with each of us being short and snapping at the other, but I sensed the call that day had resolved some unspoken rift between us. Nothing like saving a life to make two people forget their differences and come together.

"Nice work on getting that Versed onboard early," Joel said, his version of an apology.

And mine: "Good call on using the winch cable. That definitely saved his life."

Joel asked if he could buy me a coffee.

"Sure," I replied. "And I'll drive home."

That night, we hosted a big party at Casa de Medicos. All of my roommates and their girlfriends were there. Noah was dating Brooke, a visiting physician's assistant student from North Carolina who was interning at the medical clinic. Ben was hanging out with Abby, who worked on the Bear Brigade management team, studying the bruins and trying to reduce human-bear conflicts. Tami was Joel's girlfriend. She'd spent the summer as a Valley SAR siter but was now living in Bishop, California and spending the winter months bouldering. Luke was dating a ranger named Mindy, who worked in the public information office. Along with communicating with the press, she also handled the park's Instagram and Facebook feeds and answered questions like, *Where are the cages for the deer?* and *Do they turn off the waterfalls at night?* and *Where is the best place to see bison?*

"Bison are in Yellowstone, not Yosemite," she'd type, just as someone else would ask, *Where is Old Faithful?*

We had a good laugh but knew, with there being 419 National Park Service sites, it was often confusing.

Suddenly, someone tapped me on the shoulder. "Hey!"

I turned just in time to catch the beer that Brad Miller, the PA, tossed me.

I shook his hand firmly. His quarantine period from having worked with Ebola patients had ended, and he'd been given a clean bill of health.

"Thanks," I replied, cracking open a can of Pabst Blue Ribbon and taking a swig.

Following a feast, we sat around the campfire, swapping stories about crazy 9-1-1 calls. The rock climbers in the group planned future routes and trips to the Porch Swing.

"We need to get you on some rock," said Luke, turning to me. "You have climbing shoes?"

"No," I replied.

Noah said he had some I could borrow.

"Sign me up!"

I gazed around the campfire, supremely happy. After struggling during the onboarding process, I felt like I had finally been accepted by the valley shift.

And then I ran my first search-and-rescue mission, and everything fell apart.

THINKING OUTSIDE THE BOX

IN THOSE HIGH SIERRAS, I had the honor of working with—and learning from—one of the most elite rescue teams on the planet: Yosemite Search and Rescue. YOSAR, a division of Visitor and Resource Protection, was created in the late 1960s to address the increasing number of highly complex backcountry and climbing emergencies that occurred within the park. Today, YOSAR typically responds to up to 250 search-and-rescue missions a year, which range from missing-person incidents to rock-climbing falls, medical emergencies, lost hikers, and swift-water rescues.

YOSAR is comprised of Yosemite Valley and Tuolumne Meadow NPS operational staff, along with on-call summer search-and-rescue (SAR) volunteers. These SAR siters are given a tent-cabin or campsite in the valley or in Tuolumne in exchange for being on-call and assisting with emergencies. The volunteers I met had a variety of medical training and backgrounds, but they shared one common denominator: they were all amazing athletes and expert alpinists, highly trained in rock climbing, mountaineering, rope and swift-water rescue, backcountry navigation, and survival.

My first introduction to YOSAR came when Noah brought me to the SAR Cache, a rustic cabin bursting with radios, computers, and climbing gear.

"During a mission, you'll use the call sign 'SAR Grange' on the radio," Noah explained, handing me a climbing helmet, a head-lamp, a black chest harness for my radio, a pair of "approach shoes" with extra-sticky soles for good grip on slippery rocks, and a flu-orescent yellow Yosemite Search and Rescue T-shirt and jacket. Noah explained I'd wear this gear on every SAR to make sure I was safe and easily identifiable from the air or ground. As I tried on the gear, it was easy to imagine myself dangling from a helicopter, performing a daring rescue on a cliffside.

Next, Noah introduced me to two of the founding members of YOSAR, Mason Prentiss and Arthur Briggs. I shook their hands—still calloused from years of climbing—and was excited to go on my first SAR, hoping to continue their legacy of excellence.

Mason Prentiss had been a member of YOSAR since 1974 and was renowned for having the most ascents of a perilous route called Astroman on a rock spire known as Washington Column. Prentiss was also sometimes best recognized as the shirtless, wild-haired climber holding a boombox stereo while free-soloing Reeds Pinnacle in a legendary photo from the 1970s that also appears in the documentary *Valley Uprising*.

With his calm eyes and short-cropped gray hair neatly parted to the side, Arthur Briggs was more unassuming but no less accomplished. He'd arrived in Yosemite in 1970 with a physics degree from the Massachusetts Institute of Technology and was like the John Nash—the famous mathematician—of search and rescue. Briggs' own "beautiful mind" had forever changed big-wall

THINKING OUTSIDE THE BOX

helicopter rescues and search-and-rescue techniques by creating a system in which rescuers could send supplies, food, water, and communications from a helicopter to injured climbers via a nylon line and bean bag.

Briggs had also used his mathematical prowess to save countless lives by creating statistical probabilities and algorithms of where lost hikers might be found based upon their itinerary, last known location, topography, and time last seen. Briggs had been involved in almost every big SAR mission for the last forty years and had been honored by the NPS for decades of superior service. But perhaps his most miraculous rescue occurred in 1982.

On the afternoon of Sunday, January 3, Tyler Higgins, his wife, Michele, and her ten-year-old son from a previous marriage, Carl Pondella, had hopped aboard their small private plane at Mammoth–June Lake Airport. They were flying home to the Bay Area after visiting family in Oklahoma for the holidays, and this was their last refueling stop.

Just after 3:30 PM, the single-engine Grumman Tiger lifted into the sky, and the meditative hum of the motor quickly lulled Carl to sleep. Higgins's original flight plan, to fly the shortest route over the twelve-thousand-foot peaks just north of Tioga Pass, had been denied by flight control in Tonopah, Nevada, who warned that a jet stream over the Pacific Ocean was funneling two weather fronts eastward; a massive storm system was brewing. So Higgins opted instead to fly north along the eastern edge of the Sierra Nevada and then cross the vast mountain range near Reno.

But forty minutes after takeoff, Higgins was radioing flight control in Oakland, saying he was losing altitude and could see the ground. Then the radio fell silent. The airplane's last known location on radar was in the vast snowy wilderness a half mile north of Tioga Lake, just outside the entrance to Yosemite.

The storm that blew in that afternoon would end up lasting three days and would be one of the largest on record to strike Northern California. As wind, rain, and snow slammed the area, trees toppled, rivers flooded, and landslides destroyed homes. A total of thirty-three people died. The Higgins family had lost contact late Sunday afternoon, but as Monday arrived, the storm raged on, and an air search was impossible. Park officials reached out to backcountry rangers Nicklas and Dana Reyher, a couple spending their winter at a cabin in Tuolumne Meadows, eight snowy miles from the airplane's last known location. The Reyhers donned their snowshoes and rescue packs and set off into the blizzard to search for the plane through waist-deep snow.

Conditions changed little on Tuesday, but by Wednesday, the skies cleared. Mono County rescuers drove a snowcat up the mountain. Navy personnel and Yosemite rangers aboard a search-and-rescue helicopter surveyed the vicinity of the plane's last known position. Their efforts turned up nothing. The aerial search area was expanded to at least a hundred square miles on Thursday, but once again, the search proved futile.

By then, it had been four days since the crash, and the odds of anyone having survived both the impact and subzero temperatures were slim.

Since the plane's emergency locator transmitter, designed to go off on impact, hadn't activated, Arthur Briggs struggled to locate the airplane on paper. As he pored over topographical maps, the flight data baffled him: the plane's last known location was west of Mono Lake, instead of east, as it should have been according to Tyler Higgins's revised flight plan. Civil Air Patrol investigators speculated that Higgins had gotten lost and had been trying to fly his way back to his revised flight plan. Finally, late on Thursday, the investigators uncovered data from the Oakland flight control logs, revealing that shortly after takeoff Higgins had requested and received permission to fly his original route—the most direct path over Yosemite.

"Today, flight information arrives quickly on Google Earth or other digital maps, and there's a whole team of radar specialists to track a missing plane," Briggs told me when discussing the search operation from the small office where he still worked from dusk till dawn, seven days a week. "Back then, I had no computer, so I had to manually plot the coordinates for the last few minutes of the flight path on a map, to try to guess what the pilot was thinking."

For Briggs, news of the revised flight plan changed everything. "The pilot's goal had changed," he explained. "We were not searching for a plane traveling north to Reno that had gotten lost but one that intended to cross the higher altitudes of Yosemite." Briggs stayed up all night plotting data, and by Friday morning, he'd narrowed the search area to a thin strip of wilderness, six miles long, from Tioga Pass north to Mount Conness. The area had been searched on Wednesday, but buoyed by this bit of new information, the helicopter team returned to it on Friday. Late that morning, they spotted a small section of the plane's tail sticking out of the snow on the steep eastern slope of 12,057-foot White Mountain.

To access the plane, the team needed both of the Reyhers' expert mountaineering skills. Dana was already aboard the helicopter, but they raced to Tuolumne to pick up Niklas, who was waiting with skis, rope-rescue gear, and shovels. The helicopter returned to the crash site, the team dropped the Reyhers off on a ridge immediately above the plane, and Dana belayed Niklas over the edge. Niklas reached the plane and began digging frantically. When his shovel hit the window, he heard a muffled cry from inside.

It was ten-year-old Carl Pondella. After five days of subzero temperatures, the boy was in shock and severely hypothermic, and his legs were badly frostbitten. Carl's mother and stepfather had died on impact, but he was alive.

The news set off a flurry of activity. As the helicopter lowered Chief Petty Officer Craig Horn, the Reyhers pulled Carl from the back window of the airplane and helped insert him into a harness and attach him to the hoist line. As they did, the boy's eyes rolled into the back of his head, and he lost consciousness.

Carl regained consciousness in the helicopter, and JP Klein, a naval flight surgeon, was able to stabilize him until they arrived at a hospital in Fresno. There, Carl met his father and stepmother, Wade and Holly Pondella. He was later transferred to Stanford Medical Center, where doctors were forced to amputate his frostbitten legs below the knees. But four months later, Carl was recovered enough to walk out on his new prosthetic legs to throw out the first pitch at the Oakland A's season opener.

"This rescue in 1982 stands out because the odds of survival were so small, odds of finding the plane even smaller, and when we did find the plane, Carl was alive," Briggs said.

Carl Pondella went on to compete as a wrestler in high school and win a gold medal in the trick event at the World Disabled Waterski Championships in France. He now works at an orthotics and prosthetics business in Visalia that outfits new amputees, and he said in an interview that the bond he felt with his rescuers would last forever. "They taught me what it means to risk everything to save others," he said. "I can never pay them back, so I pay it forward."

After the rescue, helicopter pilot Neil Huard received the US Navy's Distinguished Flying Cross, and Craig Horn was awarded the US Navy and Marine Corps Medal, the service's second-highest non-combat award. In 2008, the Park Service gave Arthur Briggs a lifetime achievement award, and after forty-six years, he continues to work for Yosemite Search and Rescue.

· · · · · · ·

In the weeks that followed, I quickly learned there were three types of SARs in the Sierras. The first normally occurred around dusk and typically involved hikers dialing 9-1-1 because night was approaching, they didn't have a flashlight, and their cell phones were dying. Along with not having the appropriate gear, this brand of hikers often had no idea of their location, telling dispatch things like, "We're near that big strand of trees and rocky crag," as if that narrowed it down in a national park. While we sometimes sent a ranger up to help the reporting party, those calls rarely elicited a big SAR response. Normally, the lost party found their way back down by stumbling upon the trail or joining another group and hiking down with them.

The second type of mission was for people who should have called for a SAR response earlier but elected not to. These were folks who got injured in the backcountry but miraculously hiked their way out. They'd appear at trailheads or pullouts looking like the walking dead—bruised, battered, and broken—and then call 9-1-1. "Patient stated he was hiking alone above Little Yosemite Valley yesterday when he slipped on an icy patch of the trail," I wrote in one of my patient care reports. "Victim stated he fell on his left side and tried to brace his fall with his left arm. Patient stated he lost consciousness after the fall. He noticed his left wrist might be broken and decided to turn around and seek medical attention. Near Yosemite Valley, patient stated he fell off a rock and experienced another ground-level fall. Patient stated his pack rolled down a hill, so he hiked to the Valley without his pack, slept in his car due to exhaustion, and in the morning decided to seek out medical attention by having someone call 9-1-1."

The third type was the legit SARs, where the person was lost or too ill or injured to walk out, and we launched a search-and-rescue response.

The first SAR where I was the lead patient care provider occurred in early January, when I was dispatched with Sarah, my EMS supervisor and partner on the ambulance that afternoon, to the rocks beneath Lower Yosemite Falls to attend to a thirty-two-year-old woman who'd fallen. As I called "SAR Grange" over the radio for the first time, my mind raced with worry. *How high did she fall from? Did she simply trip, or is there a medical complaint behind the injury? Is her blood sugar low? Was she severely dehydrated? Did she have a blood clot in her lungs?*

Sarah and I parked the ambulance, loaded up our bags, and started up the steep paved path. She was at the front of the gurney, and I pushed from behind yet grew exhausted after only fifty yards. I was going to have to get into much better shape just to work at Yosemite, I realized.

As we crossed the footbridge, the paved path ended abruptly, so I threw the green BLS bag over one shoulder, the orange ALS bag over the other, and grabbed the gray cardiac monitor. In my dark green NPS uniform, I looked like some ridiculous Christmas tree, decorated with EMS ornaments.

Sarah asked what I was doing.

"Going to treat my patient," I replied.

"She has an ankle injury."

I protested by providing a long list of different possible diagnoses.

Sarah rolled her eyes and said something along the lines of, "When you hear hooves, think horses, not zebras," repeating the famous quote by Dr. Theodore Woodward. "Bring only narcotics, the BLS bag, and the vacuum mattress."

Moments later, we were picking our way through the boulders, searching for our patient. The polished granite rocks were wet and slippery, and at times, I had to use all four extremities to move forward.

Just then, someone called out to us in the distance, waving. "She's over here!"

I desperately needed to stop and catch my breath, but there wasn't time. A visitor was injured and needed our help.

Claire was a freckled redhead from Vancouver, Canada, who said "Eh?" a lot. She was seated on a rock, and her left ankle was obviously deformed. Fortunately, she was easygoing and didn't seem to mind that one of the people sent to rescue her—me—was symptomatic of respiratory distress.

"Hello . . . I'm . . . a . . . paramedic . . . here . . . to . . . help . . . you," I began, severely short of breath.

Sarah just stood and watched, shaking her head. "I'll get a set of vitals."

As my breath slowly returned, I determined that Claire didn't have a medical complaint before the fall nor had she hit her head or lost consciousness. She'd simply stepped the wrong way and rolled her ankle.

"All within normal limits," Sarah said as she finished taking vitals. "What next?"

"Splint the injury," I replied confidently. "And give pain meds."

"What's your extraction plan?"

I hadn't thought about that. "Walk her maybe . . . or we can try carrying?"

Sarah said I should've called for a carryout team the moment I arrived on-scene.

I'd already forgotten one of the first important lessons I'd learned in Yellowstone: "Order big and order early."

I reached for my radio to call dispatch, but Sarah stopped me. "Already done," she said. "They're en route."

With a search-and-rescue mission, Sarah said the evacuation plan was just as important as the medicine. "In fact, getting the patient out is a treatment."

As we waited for the team to arrive, Sarah and I splinted Claire's ankle and gave her an intranasal spray of Fentanyl for pain.

"Works quite fast, eh?" Claire said.

Presently, the carryout team arrived, racing up the gray rocks in their bright yellow shirts like lean, light-footed mountain goats. I was a runt among thoroughbreds. Unlike me, they all arrived calm, cool, and composed, ready to work.

"Let's place her on the vacuum mattress and move her to the gurney," I said.

The SAR team quickly went to work, readying the vacuum mattress and assisting Claire onto it. Next, they used a foot pump to remove the air, which caused the bag to conform rigidly to her body.

"Cozy, eh?" Claire said, the Fentanyl kicking in. "Maybe I'll just take a nap."

"OK, we'll lift on my count," said Joel, who'd responded on his day off to assist with the carryout. "Is anyone not ready?"

"Actually, we'll lift on my count," I said, interjecting.

Joel informed me he was at Claire's head and, therefore, would make the call.

"Yes, but she's my patient," I countered.

"Fine," said Joel, backing off. "Your call."

The team lifted on my command, and we carried her through the rocks to the gurney, pausing for team members to reset or switch out when they grew tired. I was trying to stay connected to Claire and her complaint while also directing the team, and it all felt disjointed and awkward. Worst of all, I felt as if I'd angered

Joel and the rest of the YOSAR members, possibly compromising the valley-shift rapport I'd spent weeks building.

The rest of the call went well. We started an IV on Claire, gave her pain medication intravenously, and transferred her to Mercy Ambulance at El Portal. But driving back into the valley that night, I scribbled down improvement areas: *Get in better shape, form an extrication plan sooner, delegate specific jobs to my crew to avoid role confusion.* The patient compartment of the ambulance was often referred to as "the box"; for me to become an effective SAR team member, I needed to learn how to think outside of it.

Sarah also suggested I focus on the medical aspects of future calls and designate a litter captain— one specific person to lead the team in evacuating the patient from the environment.

"You can do that?" I asked. In LA, I had to run all aspects of the call, but it was different out here in the wild.

Sarah said I *should* do that.. "Those guys are experts at patient packaging, rope rescue, and extrication," she explained. "Joel is always a great choice. He was attempting to do that, and you stood him down."

"He probably hates me now, huh?" I worried.

Sarah laughed. "He may seem stern, but he's really just a softie on the inside," she explained. "But you might apologize next time you see him."

Sarah added that I should keep a "go bag" in the ambulance with the ten essentials for hiking: sunscreen, extra clothing, compass, sunglasses, headlamp, a multitool, matches, a map, extra water, and food.

"When you go on a SAR, you never know if you'll be gone for two hours or two days," Sarah commented. "Plus, it's good to have that stuff on the ambulance in case we're running calls all day."

While she appreciated that I was being thorough with my laundry list of potential diagnoses, she explained, "It's not feasible to carry all the equipment with you on a SAR because it's cumbersome, slows you down, and then you risk being injured. Rather than focus on all the things it could be, deal with what you know and only bring what you need."

• • • • • • •

I was ravenous by the time Sarah and I drove back into the valley, but there wasn't time to eat. Another SAR had dropped while we were transporting Claire out of the park to El Portal. A twenty-eight-year-old man from Paris named Henrie, who only spoke *un peu* English, had slipped on some ice on the Upper Falls Trail, near Yosemite Point, and slid twenty feet down a steep rock face.

Luke and another ranger had formed a hasty team and hiked to the patient. A hasty team is often employed in the early hours of a search and rescue. The goal is to send a small group with minimal gear to rapidly locate the patient while they are still alive and then determine what additional medical and evacuation resources are needed to complete the mission.

Once on scene, Luke's team found Henrie complaining of abdominal pain, pelvic pain, and a broken leg. Due to the fading sunlight and the possibility that Henrie was bleeding out into his pelvis, they requested a short-haul rescue. A California Highway Patrol (CHP) helicopter flew to the area and lowered a litter. Luke and another ranger quickly packaged Henrie in a vacuum mattress and secured him to the litter, and with Luke attached, the bird lifted.

Sarah informed me our job on that call was to meet the CHP helicopter at Ahwahnee Meadow, stabilize the patient, and then transfer him to a life flight helicopter with medical supplies and a critical care team that would stabilize him further and transport him to a trauma center in Fresno.

As we arrived at Ahwahnee Meadow, we found the CHP helo already on the ground, so we quickly unfastened Henrie from the hoist line and carried him in the vacuum mattress to our gurney.

I wanted to make a connection with Henrie, so I told him I'd studied French in high school. "Je parle français. Je l'ai étudié au lycée."

Of course, he then assumed I was fluent and went off. "J'ai mal à l'estomac," he winced. "Avez-vous quelque chose pour la douleur? Pouvez-vous me rassurer? Puis-je appeler ma femme?"

"Je parle *un peu* français," I replied, stressing the *little* part. In the back of the ambulance, I worked fast—starting an IV and giving Henrie pain medication—to wash away my errors on the last call. I also applied low-flow oxygen since Henrie was uncomfortable when he inhaled deeply.

Sarah and I performed a physical assessment. Henrie's body was in rough shape. He'd likely broken a few ribs, cracked the bowl of his pelvis, and busted his lower leg. Since I was lead on the last call, Sarah took primary and selected "falling from a high place" in the dropdown menu of her patient care report when it asked about the cause of the injury.

Sarah was right. Yosemite definitely was a "trauma park."

Due to the late hour, the life flight helicopter elected to do a hot load, meaning they'd keep the rotors spinning, as we transferred Henrie to their care.

"Safe travels, Henrie," I said. "Bon voyage."

"Merci," he replied, shaking my hand.

• • • • • • •

In the days that followed, I vowed to get in better shape. My goal was to become what Lt. Col. Stephen Rush, MD, a flight surgeon and the former medical director for the US Air Force's elite pararescue team, termed a "professional rescue athlete."

I committed to eating healthier, joined my roommates at the employee gym in Curry Village to lift weights, and attended the free yoga class at the wellness center every Wednesday night. But my main objective was improving my cardiovascular shape. I was ashamed at my breathless, sweaty presentation to Claire on my first SAR mission.

I vowed to get in better shape by running the trail up to Yosemite Falls. At first, I could barely make it to Columbia Point, at one mile and one-thousand feet up, but as the weeks passed, I was able to scramble all 2,700 feet up the steep switchbacks to stand triumphantly over the Upper Falls—North America's tallest waterfall. I was pleased with my progress, but I wasn't working out for myself so much as for that distant day when I had to get to victims trapped on the upper floor of a burning building or having a heart attack far up a rocky trail. Instead of having to catch my breath when I reached them, my goal was to be able to focus all my energy on saving their lives.

• • • • • • •

It was an unseasonably warm winter that year, and the guys from Casa de Medicos and I would occasionally play hoops at the basketball courts in front of the Yosemite Elementary School. We were in a spirited game on January 25, when Anthony Stanton, twenty-four, rappelled off the end of his rope and felt himself falling through midair. He was climbing a popular route known as Royal Arches, due to its high cliff bands and granite exfoliation arches.

As the tones dropped, we raced to the ambulance parked beside the basketball court and drove toward the SAR Cache. Along with saving a life, I also hoped to redeem myself as a SAR member, but the radio traffic sounded grim.

"I have eyes on him," Luke, who was standing at the bottom of the route with binoculars, announced over the radio. "He landed on a ledge, and I have no movement."

"Keep watching," ordered Sarah, incident commander for this emergency.

"Still no movement," Luke said again.

Dispatch informed us that the reporting party, his climbing buddy, estimated Anthony had fallen over five hundred feet.

"Nothing."

Sarah had Luke form a hasty team with another climbing ranger and scale the cliff face. That's where they found Anthony, deceased.

It was too late in the evening to bring his body down from the ledge, so they covered him with tarps and secured them in place.

The following morning, Noah and I parked the ambulance to block the entrance to the trail leading to Royal Arches. Our job was to hold a perimeter so no "lookie-loos" got through. We placed bright orange signs at the trailhead that said, "Rescue in Progress," but sadly, we knew it was only a recovery.

Anthony's family drove out from Stockton, California, to receive the body. Anthony loved climbing. He'd served in the army and was studying computer-aided drafting and design.

Even though Noah and I hadn't been directly involved with the recovery, his family shook our hands and, through tears, thanked us for bringing their boy home.

16

SCOPE OF PRACTICE

AS A PARAMEDIC with the National Park Service, I was lucky enough to have the kind of expanded scope of practice rarely allowed in an urban setting, where the hospitals were a short drive away. I realized this on my sixth call in Yosemite, when we were dispatched to the Upper Pines Campground for a woman with a dislocated shoulder.

Fifteen minutes earlier, Kaitlin Hopgood—a twenty-four-year-old student at the San Francisco Art Institute who wore all-black everything—had been walking near her campsite when she'd tripped, landing on her outstretched right arm. Her shoulder slipped from its socket, and she had immediate and severe pain.

We found her seated on the ground, recoiling in severe distress, with an indentation where her right humeral head—the top of her arm bone—should have been.

Ben, Luke, and I quickly assessed her injury and took a set of vital signs. By then, it was after 7:00 pm, and the medical clinic was closed.

"On a scale of one to ten," Ben asked Kaitlin, "how would you rate your pain?"

"A twenty," she replied, wincing. "Help me."

When Ben informed Kaitlin he'd like to give her pain medication and take her to the closest hospital—over an hour away—she declined. "I'm in school. There's no way I can afford that," she managed. "Can't you just pop it back in?"

I glanced over at Ben who was the team lead. "Thoughts?"

Ben handed me the cell phone we kept on the ambulance. "Give Dr. Groves a call and get his thoughts."

Dr. Groves was the physician at the clinic and our medical director. He was a graduate of Vanderbilt University School of Medicine and had spent the last few years living in the valley with his family. He also truly believed in the competency and life-saving abilities of paramedics.

When I got him on the line, Dr. Groves told me he was out of the valley. "But you can go ahead and give her Fentanyl for pain and reduce her shoulder," he directed.

This directive meant we could pop her dislocated shoulder back into place.

"If she has no other complaints and still doesn't want to go to the hospital by ambulance, she can refuse," Dr. Groves continued. "However, I'd still recommend she go on her own."

"Copy," I replied nonchalantly, before the weight of Dr. Groves's words actually registered. "Wait, what?"

Dr. Groves repeated himself and then told us to call him back if we had any additional questions.

"Will do," I replied.

I passed Dr. Groves's thoughts along to Ben and Luke, who in turn explained them to Kaitlin. She quickly consented to treatment, and we had her sit on a log to give us more room to work.

Ben sprayed a dose of Fentanyl up Kaitlin's right nostril, as Luke readied himself beside her shoulder.

Watching them, my mind raced with worry: *What if Kaitlin had an adverse reaction to the Fentanyl? What if we reduced her shoulder wrong and caused tendon damage?* Then I asked myself the bigger, more pressing question: *What if I stopped the self-limiting thoughts and instead honored the paramedic training we'd all received and Dr. Groves's belief in us and simply got the job done?*

"Let me know how I can help," I said to Ben.

"Will do," he replied. "Just waiting for the Fentanyl to kick in."

When Kaitlin stated she could feel her pain subside, Ben and Luke began the shoulder reduction. Luke massaged Kaitlin's neck and shoulder to lessen the muscle spasms, and Ben applied gentle downward traction to her right arm.

As Kaitlin winced in pain, I coached her breathing. "In through your nose for a count of three and out through your mouth for a count of six."

Luke continued massaging, as Ben slowly performed an external rotation of her arm while applying gentle downward traction.

"Deep breaths," I said. "You're doing great."

Suddenly, Kaitlin's shoulder popped back into the socket, giving her instant relief.

"Ahh, so much better!" she said, smiling.

Following the reduction, we took another set of vital signs and verified that Kaitlin didn't have an altered mental status from the Fentanyl and had a good pulse and blood flow in her right arm. Her follow-up plan of care would be to have her boyfriend—a tall, skinny guy with a chain wallet and hoops in his ears—drive her to John C. Fremont Hospital in Mariposa for additional evaluation.

Kaitlin signed the necessary refusal paperwork, and as we walked back to the ambulance, I decided that being a remote, wilderness paramedic was the most challenging, dynamic, and best job in the world.

· · · · · · ·

Despite knowing the treatment protocols at Yosemite and having Dr. Groves's encouragement, it took me some time to become comfortable with my new freedom. In hindsight, my conservative approach manifested in potentially undertreating pain, recommending full spinal precautions when they probably weren't needed, or suggesting to patients that they go to the hospital when I knew, deep down, it likely wasn't necessary.

I resolved to be a more confident, critical-thinking medic. This was my new attitude when Noah and I approached a car parked at Curry Village one evening.

"Hi, sir," I began. "What's the problem today?"

"I can't stop throwing up," the man said, pausing to do just that in the wheel well.

Shaun Newitt, thirty, worked "two weeks on, two weeks off" in the oil fields of Bakersfield. He told me he was in good shape but had taken a twenty-mile hike that day with a six-thousand-foot change in elevation each way. He went "extra hard and extra fast and didn't drink too much water."

There was a lot I wanted to check out, but first I needed to get Shaun out of the backseat of this car, where he was vomiting into a wrinkled plastic grocery bag.

"Can we move into the ambulance so my partner and I can check you out?"

"Anything," he said, pausing to wretch, "just help me feel better."

We assisted Shaun into the ambulance and began assessing him. Based on his strenuous day, poor fluid intake, and reports of dark-colored urine, it was simple to assume he was severely dehydrated and, possibly, experiencing rhabdomyolysis, a potentially lethal condition where toxins from muscle breakdown entered the bloodstream, causing organ failure. But, as I'd been taught in paramedic school, I would confirm my suspicion by eliminating all other possibilities.

Noah and I jumped into assessment mode. By then we'd run so many calls together, we hardly needed to talk. We were performing a grand choreography, so when Shaun started to retch again, Noah was there with a blue emesis bag to catch the yellow bile before it covered the gurney and my uniform.

We checked Shaun's vital signs, heart rhythm, and blood sugar, inquired about his medical history and, in the process, essentially ruled out many possible causes for his nausea and vomiting: a heart attack, diabetic emergency, GI bleed, traumatic brain bleed, bowel obstruction, drugs or alcohol, appendicitis, acute gastroenteritis, and even hyponatremia, a rare condition where you can die from drinking too much water due to low levels of sodium in the body. The condition was most often seen in hot, dry environments (like the Grand Canyon) where hikers consumed an excess amount of water, flushing all the electrolytes from their system.

Noah placed an IV, and we gave Shaun Zofran for nausea, then hung a bag of fluid and over the next thirty minutes, administered one thousand milliliters of saline. I also called medical control since Shaun was requesting not to go to the hospital and was already feeling better.

"I'm comfortable with that if you are," said Brad Miller, the physician's assistant.

Shaun's complaint may not have had the dramatic element of a cardiac arrest or major trauma, but treating a patient with nausea and vomiting could be one of my favorite calls—it was so satisfying to see someone's pain and discomfort ease before your eyes. As the Zofran and fluid worked their magic, color returned to Shaun's face, his furrowed brow relaxed, and he started to smile and tell us about himself.

"I'm actually one of the best cornhole players in the USA," he said. "Not to brag, but I crushed it last year at the Tailgator Championships in Vegas."

"That's awesome!" we told him.

Shaun said we should go next year. "And I'll buy you drinks for helping me."

By the time the IV fluid finished, Shaun felt much better. His buddies would drive him home, and he'd spend the rest of the night sipping Gatorade, having some dinner, and taking it easy, he promised.

"Sounds good," I replied. "And definitely give us a call back if your condition changes or worsens."

Later, Noah and I drove a loop around the valley. Waterfalls crashed in the distance, serenading us with their soft roar, and the Merced River sparkled in the late afternoon light. Gazing around, I felt truly happy and content. Along with the amazing people I'd met while working for the National Park Service and the breathtaking scenery, the expanded scope of practice was just one more reason I loved working as a wilderness medic. But I wondered what it all meant for my dream of returning to Los Angeles.

17

FREQUENT FLYERS

SOME PATIENTS DIAL 9-1-1 SO OFTEN that they ought to get frequent flyer miles. Leroy, the concession employee who'd suffered a skull fracture during my first week at Yosemite, became our frequent-flyer. After he returned from the hospital in Fresno, he called us for constipation, a bad headache, and of course, more seizures. In fact, he dialed 9-1-1 so often that Noah and I named a diagnosis after him one afternoon, when we were dispatched to Curry Village for a fifty-five-year-old male having convulsions.

"Think it's Leroy having a seizure?" I asked, as we wheeled the gurney to his front door.

Noah nodded. "It's definitely a *Leizure*."

Sure enough, it was our Leroy. He'd been clearing dishes and cleaning tables when he started seizing, fell backward, and hit his head. He quickly regained consciousness and, despite our best attempts, refused our offer to transport him to the hospital.

"I'm concerned about you," I said. "You really should be seen by a doctor."

Leroy shook his head no. "Thanks for the offer, but I feel fine and want to stay here."

Since Leroy was alert, oriented, and answering our questions appropriately, we couldn't force him to go. I suggested Leroy take the rest of the day off and told him to call us back anytime.

"Will do," he replied, grabbing a hand towel to continue wiping down tables.

As we cleared the scene, I worried a seizure would kill Leroy one day. I knew he'd be safer living in an assisted living facility in Fresno with nurses on duty and beds with padded rails. However, Yellowstone's "bucket listers" had shown me how, at a certain point in one's life, living better became more important than living longer. To move Leroy from the valley would be the equivalent of taking him off life support; he'd wither away. His life had meaning and purpose at Yosemite. Each morning, he walked outside and said hello to his "neighbors"—Cathedral Peak, Clouds Rest, and Half Dome, as Yosemite Falls thundered in the distance. Then he walked to Curry Village where he spent the day clearing dishes and washing tables. Leroy's life here had beauty, meaning, and purpose. You could see it in his dedication to his job and the way he instructed families to say "Cheese!" when they asked him to take their picture. Given Leroy's lengthy medical history, I always encouraged him to go to the hospital, but it was only so he could get healthy and return to his happy place: Yosemite.

Along with frequent-flyer patients, we also responded to frequent addresses. After working in Yosemite for a few weeks, I decided the ice-skating rink at Curry Village was one such place. We responded to the "trauma rink" daily—and occasionally, multiple times a day—for injured ice skaters with forehead lacerations, busted noses, or bruised cheekbones. The falls at the rink always seemed to end in mild complaints such as sprained ankles, strained wrists, or head bumps, which were typically the result of adults' trying to play the ice-skating game "crack the whip" with their kids.

So when Noah and I were dispatched to the ice rink one Saturday, we weren't expecting anything too serious. If you respond to a homeless guy in the alley who is just drunk five days in a row, or the elderly lady who repeatedly activates her medical alert alarm by accident at 3:00 AM, or the four-hundred-pound man who simply needs to be helped off the toilet a few times each week, you get lulled into a routine. Running these calls hour after hour, day after day, the evidence stacks up. Everything points to the same verdict: not serious. You are no longer suspicious when you hear a particular address or patient's name. Without realizing it, you are caught in a rip current of complacency. Who was to say that today wasn't the day the homeless man was having a diabetic emergency instead of being intoxicated, or that the woman with the medical alert bracelet was actually having a heart attack?

"This is our second run to the ice rink today," I said as we parked and radioed dispatch that we were on-scene.

"I think it's our third," Noah replied. "Or maybe that was yesterday. It's all a blur."

I was lead and instructed Noah to grab the basic life support bag and laptop computer. I was sure this call was going to result in a patient refusal like all the others. As we wheeled the gurney toward a woman on the ice—doing our best not to slip—I was ready for anything but not expecting to need to be.

When we approached, I noticed the woman sitting on the ice in mild distress. She was conscious and breathing, but she looked dazed. There was a small puddle of yellow vomit in front of her.

I knelt next to her, quickly introduced myself, and assessed her mental status. "What's your name?"

"Veronica," she said anxiously.

"Can you tell me where you are right now?"

"Yosemite National Park."

Behind me, Noah obtained some information about her medical history from her boyfriend, Doug.

"Can you tell me what happened, Veronica?" I continued.

"I fell," she managed, her eyes scanning the rink like searchlights.

Veronica was also able to tell me the correct date and the name of our current president, so I determined she was alert and oriented.

"Did you lose consciousness?"

"She was out for a good three minutes and then threw up once," Doug chimed in.

Was it really three minutes? I thought to myself. *Or was Doug overestimating the time?* That was often the case with family members and friends in an emergency.

Veronica's pupils—always a good window into a patient's neurological function—were equal and reactive, and as I palpated her neck and spine, I found no obvious trauma. She denied feeling any pain. Since she'd hit her head in the fall, I was going to recommend she go to the hospital for a CT scan.

I suspected a mild concussion. But a moment later, I felt her pulse and discovered it was rapid and weak. And her skin was pale and felt cool and dry. My mind quickly filled with questions: *Was she still spooked from her fall? Mildly hypothermic from sitting on the ice? Or was she going into shock? Had she suffered a mild concussion or a major traumatic brain injury? Could this type of fall—which for many previous patients had yielded only mild complaints—have suddenly turned deadly?*

There was no way to tell out there on the ice, in the fading sun and winter wind, so Noah and I loaded Veronica onto the gurney and moved her into the back of the ambulance. Doug followed, sitting down in the captain's seat behind the gurney.

In the ambulance, we blasted the heat and removed Veronica's black down jacket and pink gloves so we could better assess her.

"A set of vital signs and blood sugar," I said to Noah, who quickly went to work.

I rechecked Veronica's head for any blood, deformities, or depressions on her skull but didn't find any visible trauma. By then, the patient compartment of the ambulance was bright and warm, yet Veronica's anxiety about her fall wasn't lessening. She was still shivering and breathing at a quick clip. Beads of sweat dotted her forehead.

"I'm going to throw up," she suddenly blurted. "I'm going to throw up!"

I grabbed a blue emesis bag from the cabinet and handed it to her.

"I'm going to throw up! I'm going to throw up!" she repeated in rapid-fire succession.

Veronica didn't get sick, so I tried to calm her and lower her heart and respiratory rate. "Ma'am, try to relax and lengthen your breath," I offered. "We're going to take good care of you."

"I'm going to throw up!" she said again, frantically.

Noah set down the blood pressure cuff and stethoscope and relayed Veronica's vital signs. With the exception of her heart rate, they were all within normal limits.

"What do you want to do?" he asked.

The challenge of being a wilderness paramedic was having to make split-second decisions about patient care with limited equipment, knowing your choice might alter the course of a patient's life forever. Unlike a doctor in the ER—or an urban EMS provider—we couldn't call a neurologist or cardiologist for a consult or just rush patients to the nearest hospital a few blocks away. There was no safety net in remote medicine and nothing to hide behind. You were alone out there in the wild. The treatment protocols were written on the page in black and white, but the job was a hazy shade of gray.

"What shall we do?" Noah asked again, checking his watch.

I pondered the options. The closest medical facility, apart from the small clinic in Yosemite Valley, was forty-five minutes away. It was a small community hospital. They had a CT scanner, but if they found anything critical, they weren't equipped to do anything about it. The city of Fresno had the closest trauma center, but that was two hours away by ground or half an hour by helicopter.

I gazed down at Veronica, still anxious, breathing rapidly, and looking pale, cool, and clammy.

"Ma'am, where are we right now?" I asked, rechecking her mental status.

"I'm going to throw up. I'm going to throw up," she said again, arms flailing.

"What year is it?"

Veronica didn't answer.

I turned to Noah. "Launch a helicopter now."

"You sure?" he asked.

"Really?" Doug asked. "A helicopter? Isn't that a little excessive?"

I hadn't expected this resistance, and, for a moment, I questioned myself. I turned back to Veronica. "Ma'am, can you tell me where you are right now?"

"I'm going to throw up—"

I'd read about epidural brain bleeds years ago in my EMT school textbook. Patients hit their head and lose consciousness, after which they undergo a lucid interval when they appear fine, alert, and oriented. However, as arterial bleeding from the initial impact begins to put pressure on the brain, their mental status deteriorates, and if they aren't rushed to the hospital, breathing and other vital functions begin to shut down, leading to an anoxic brain injury and cardiac arrest. I'd also read about epidural brain bleeds in the paper when actress Natasha Richardson fell while skiing on a beginner's trail in 2009. She was initially fine, joking about the incident and ignoring the insistent pleas from ski patrol that she go to a doctor. Two days later, she was dead.

"I'm going to throw up! I'm going to throw up!" Veronica blurted again.

"Launch the helicopter," I said, relying on the one vital sign no blood-pressure cuff or cardiac monitor could measure—my gut instinct. "She's not answering my questions. She has an altered mental state and is getting worse."

As I performed another rapid trauma exam and pulled out my IV supplies, Noah radioed in our request, then turned to me. "Medevac has launched. ETA thirty minutes."

Yosemite dispatch summoned firefighters and a fire engine to help us secure the landing zone in the field across from the medical clinic, and Luke, who'd arrived on-scene, hopped in the front seat to drive.

"Tell me when you're ready," he said, peering back in the rearview mirror.

"Drive!" Noah and I shouted in unison.

Luke hit the emergency lights, activated the sirens, and pulled out. I instructed Noah to monitor Veronica's airway and breathing as I applied some electrodes to look at her heart rhythm and monitor her blood pressure.

The minutes that followed could have sent chills up the spine of even the most seasoned paramedic. Veronica's level of consciousness continued to decline, her eyes rolled into the upper corner of their sockets, and her breathing became deep and slow. She'd occasionally wake and mumble, "I'm going to throw up!" before drifting off again.

When Noah took vital signs again, her blood pressure was starting to rise, and her heart rate was slowing down, which, in conjunction with her irregular respirations, told us the intracranial pressure in her skull was starting to rise and she could have a seizure or go into cardiac arrest at any minute.

Veronica maintained her gag reflex, which meant we couldn't attempt to put a breathing tube in her windpipe lest she would start throwing up and choke on her vomit. Instead, we placed a nasopharyngeal airway into her right nostril. This thin, rubber, trumpet-shaped device would help prevent her tongue from sealing off her airway.

"I can't believe this is happening," Doug said in shock as we arrived at the landing zone.

In time, we heard the rhythmic whoosh of rotary blades and a helo landing. Moments later, a flight nurse and paramedic hopped in the back of the ambulance.

"What do you have?" the nurse asked.

"Thirty-seven-year-old female with an altered mental status, secondary to hitting her head while ice skating. She had a lucid interval on-scene, but her mentation quickly altered," I said. "Possible epidural bleed."

The nurse scribbled notes, then attempted to rouse Veronica, first by calling her name and then by giving her a strong sternal rub with her knuckle. Nothing. The nurse lifted Veronica's eyelid to assess her pupils, then quickly turned to her partner: "She needs to be intubated before we leave," she said quickly.

With that, she and her partner quickly sedated Veronica and inserted a breathing tube in her windpipe as Noah and I obtained a second IV in her other arm. By then, we had moved Doug outside in order to give us more room to work. He stood sadly outside, staring at the ambulance with a blank, traumatized expression. Moments later, Veronica's airway secured, she was hooked up to a ventilator, delivering one breath every six seconds, and we moved her to the helicopter.

"Move back!" I warned some tourists, snapping pictures. "There's gonna be a lot of wind and debris flying when this thing launches."

The pilot started the engine and rotors kicked up dust. The helicopter lifted slowly and tentatively, as if unsure of its wings, and then rose higher before shifting into high gear and disappearing over Half Dome.

Luke summoned dispatch on the radio. "Life flight has lifted and you can show all fire and EMS units clear of scene."

With that, all the emergency vehicles left and life in Yosemite Valley returned to normal. But not for Veronica and certainly not for me.

• • • • • • •

The flight nurse called later that evening. "Great job," she began, her voice echoing in the helicopter hangar. "Veronica had a skull fracture and an epidural bleed. You nailed it!"

"Thanks," I managed.

While perhaps I should have shared her excitement at a job well done, I felt sick to my stomach. Early in my career, I took great pleasure when I nailed a difficult diagnosis or procedure like placing an IV or inserting a breathing tube into the trachea. But as the years went by, the thrill of these interventions wore off. Now I was more concerned with what was really important: the patient's outcome. It wasn't about what interventions I could do to my patients but how they fared after my treatment. Would Veronica ever open her eyes? Would her neurological status ever return to normal? Would she ever ice skate again or return to being the person who she'd been before?

I wanted answers, but all I heard were leaves rattling in the wind, as tree branches cast crooked shadows on the snow.

18

MEDITATION AT GUNPOINT

I TIGHTENED THE LEG LOOPS OF MY HARNESS, took a deep breath, and gazed up at the granite slab before me.

"Here goes nothing," I said, reaching for the wall and placing my right foot on my first toe hold. "Climbing!"

"Climb on!" Noah replied.

As my climbing partner who stayed on the ground as I climbed, Noah's job was to manage the rope—feeding more when I yelled "Slack!" and tightening when I shouted "Take!"—but his most important duty was to engage the belay device when I fell (which I most certainly would, since it was my first time rock climbing). And once I'd topped out, or was too stuck or too tired to continue, Noah would then lower me to the ground.

I scrambled to the top of a few boulders at the approach and then started up the wall, locking my fingers on a handhold and jamming my foot into a slanting crack.

"Nice," Noah encouraged. "Keep your body close to the wall and use your legs."

When I'd arrived in Yosemite in November, I'd quickly learned that residing in the valley meant living at the center of the rock-climbing world. You could see it in the self-proclaimed "climbing bums" at historic Camp 4, who were tackling Midnight Lightning, the world's most famous bouldering route, and in the appearance of Alex Honnold—the famed free-soloist who had climbed the world's tallest rock faces without any ropes or safety gear—at a potluck at a fellow park ranger's place one night.

"He's here!" I texted Noah one rainy night. "Get to lower housing now!"

You could see it in the Dark Wizard himself, Dean Potter, slacklining high above Yosemite Falls—and in a conversation I had with a woman named Lynn at El Capitan Meadow one January afternoon.

Dozens of us had gathered to watch renowned climbers Tommy Caldwell and Kevin Jorgeson attempting what was widely known as the most difficult ascent in rock climbing: the Dawn Wall on El Capitan. The Dawn Wall was like a frozen river of granite, with only the tiniest of fissures and cracks, that rose three thousand feet from the valley floor to the summit of El Capitan. Caldwell and Jorgeson would employ only their arms and legs to make the ascent—a process known as free climbing. While they had ropes, they were to be used only to catch them if they fell. The climb generated strong media buzz, and every afternoon over the course of their nineteen-day push, Noah and I would drive our ambulance out to the meadow across from El Capitan to join the dozens of journalists, tourists, and rock climbing fans charting the men's progress with binoculars and spotting scopes.

"Welcome to Yosemite," I said to one of the female spectators, assuming a host-like tone.

"Thank you," she replied.

Her name was Lynn, and she was a petite, athletic woman in her fifties with a friendly smile.

"Ever been to Yosemite before?"

She gave me an odd look. "Um, a few times."

I nodded in the direction of Jorgeson and Caldwell high up on El Cap, tiny dots floating in a sea of granite. "Amazing!" I said. "You ever rock climbed?"

"A bit," she replied politely.

Suddenly, Noah pulled me aside. He'd been listening a few feet away and, evidently, didn't like what he heard.

"You idiot!" he hissed discreetly. "Do you know who that is?"

"No clue."

"Lynn Hill!" he gasped, looking over my shoulder to make sure she wasn't listening.

"Who?" I asked obliviously.

"She's one of the best rock climbers ever!"

As Noah told me about Lynn's many feats—being the first person to ever make a one-day free ascent of The Nose on El Capitan, crushing dozens of other first ascents and elite routes, and being invited to the White House and on *The David Letterman Show*—I felt more than stupid. But then Noah suddenly brightened and told me there was a way I could redeem myself.

"Take my picture with her!"

Lynn—who was as humble and kind as she was accomplished—generously agreed to a photo. Afterward, we all took turns watching Jorgeson and Caldwell through the telescopic camera of legendary photographer Tom Evans. For over twenty years, Tom has authored the famous climbing blog, *El Cap Report*, which provided daily details on the epic triumphs and tragedies of rock climbing's most famous route.

Gazing up at El Cap, I couldn't help but be inspired by Caldwell and Jorgeson's determination and audacity. The pair had spent six years preparing for this climb, returning to Yosemite every fall to spend weeks scouting the route, identifying handholds, and practicing pitches. Watching them that afternoon, and seeing their portaledges—deployable hanging tents like nylon cocoons—two thousand feet in the air under gray clouds and muted sun, it occurred to me that athletes always knew when the big game would begin. And so it was with other endeavors: actors or musicians knowing their cues; astronauts counting down before launch; Navy SEALs planning for the exact moment when their team would insert into the mission site.

First responders had no such luxury. Whether working in fire, EMS, or law enforcement, when the alarm tones dropped, we never knew what we'd be dispatched to face: a pediatric cardiac arrest, a fully involved structure fire with trapped occupants, or a mass shooting. We had no idea which of our skills would be tested or when a traumatic call's horrifying sights and sounds would assault our psyches, leaving invisible but permanent tattoos. We didn't know when we would confront our own Dawn Wall.

The details surrounding Caldwell and Jorgeson's historic Dawn Wall climb were impressive, but I was most inspired by the friendship between the two men. When Jorgeson got stuck on the fifteenth pitch—a brutal, nearly impossible, traverse—Caldwell, who'd already climbed the route, didn't leave his buddy behind. Instead, he waited six days and risked the success of the entire endeavor to wait for his friend. Jorgeson eventually completed the fifteenth pitch, and the two finished the historic climb on January 14, 2015, and in the process, reaffirmed all that was good about friendship, achievement, and venturing into the great outdoors.

A similar familial bond existed among park rangers and first responders. I felt it on the ambulance, and I felt it on my first climb, as I struggled to scale a difficult route known as Highway Star with Noah and his friends.

An hour earlier, we'd parked at a small pullout on the banks of the Merced River. Like my California friends who made me paddle out into towering waves the first time I surfed, I realized veteran rock climbers like Noah took me to the walls they wanted to climb versus the beginner routes I should've learned on.

As I squeezed my feet into a borrowed pair of climbing shoes that felt three sizes too small, Noah scrambled to the top of the route, where he set up a top-rope anchor system, employing a stand of deep-rooted trees.

Highway Star was an imposing wall of immense granite "flakes" shaped like the states of Texas, California, and Idaho. I thought the crag looked unclimbable, but Noah and his buddies scaled the massive wall with ease, before lowering back to the ground and cracking celebratory beers.

I had no such luck.

"I'm stuck!" I yelled from a small rock outcropping, fifteen feet above the ground.

"You're doing great," Noah encouraged. "Jam your foot into that crack, then reach up and pinch that hold!"

"My forearms are on fire!" I lamented.

"Keep going, bro!" yelled one of Noah's friends.

Noah advised me to take a break and try to see the wall with a new set of eyes. "Lean back and let the rope hold you," he said. "I got you."

Noah's advice about avoiding tunnel vision when confronted with an obstacle felt like a good metaphor for wilderness medicine. We had to improvise, be creative, and pay attention to the numerous details of treating patients while not losing sight of the end goal: getting the patient to definitive care.

I spotted a new handhold to my left and a different route to the top. I orchestrated the move successfully, gripping with my hands and jamming my feet into tiny cracks.

Noah and his buddies cheered wildly, and I immediately fell in love with rock climbing. From my spot on the wall, the route grew steeper and widened into a large fissure. I wanted to continue, but I knew nothing about crack climbing and was quickly exhausted.

"Take!" I yelled down to Noah. "Lower!"

"You sure?"

"Lower, please!" I yelled.

"Lowering!" Noah repeated, using the same closed-loop communication technique we employed on the ambulance, where you repeated a request, or medication dosage, to prevent errors.

As I returned to the ground and untied from the rope, I pondered the intense focus and effort it took to rock climb, and the high stakes. "It's intense!"

"Like meditation at gunpoint," Noah concluded.

The phrase rang true. A week later, I was dispatched to a route known as Jam Crack for a climber who had fallen. I immediately feared the worst. Would this be a rescue? Or a body recovery?

It was my first SAR lead since my botched call beneath Lower Yosemite Falls involving the thirty-two-year old woman from Canada who'd fallen and broken her ankle, so I wanted to redeem myself. Jam Crack was only a few hundred yards from the medical clinic, so we arrived quickly.

I was lead patient-care provider on the call, meaning I would make all of the medical decisions and assign tasks, such as obtaining a set of vital signs and splinting, to my team. It was important to have one designated "lead" so everyone wasn't talking to the patient at once and people didn't start "freelancing," the term given to individuals who branched off from the group and worked

independently—doing what they wanted, when they wanted—
often to the detriment of the overall mission.

As we pulled up, I saw bystanders in the distance crouched
around a climber lying supine below a vertical rock wall. "He's
alive!"

I immediately told dispatch to request a search-and-rescue
team to assist us. "We'll do basic life support on-scene and
advanced life support en route to the hospital," I told Noah as
we pulled up. I'd decided that a prebrief before a call was just as
important as the debrief after. It allowed my team to know their
roles and responsibilities, prevented role confusion, and gave us
the opportunity to visualize successful implementation as we traveled toward our patient.

"Copy," Noah replied. "What equipment do you want?"

Remembering the motto, "When you hear hoofbeats, think
horses, not zebras," I told Noah to grab only the BLS bag, vacuum
mattress, and narcotics.

We found Otto Weber lying at the base of the wall. He was a
twenty-eight-year-old tourist from Germany with deep blue eyes
and prematurely graying hair. As I approached, I knew Otto was
conscious, had a patent airway, and could breathe because he was
arguing with his girlfriend.

"What were you thinking?" he asked in a thick German accent,
wincing in pain.

"Sorry for this!" replied his girlfriend, Inge, with an equally
thick German accent.

"We went over how to belay!"

"Sorry!"

Otto's head was being held in neutral-alignment by a bystander
named Maggie, who informed me that she'd taken a Wilderness
First Aid class from National Outdoor Leadership School (NOLS).
Maggie updated me on the accident: Otto had been climbing about

ten feet up when he fell. Inge hadn't been paying attention on the belay device, so she'd failed to engage her brake hand. The rope then whipped through the belay device, and Otto crashed to the ground. He didn't lose consciousness but landed directly on his feet.

"Chief complaint is bilateral ankle pain and back pain," Maggie announced, giving me a quick patient report. "No remarkable medical history."

I introduced myself to Otto and told him I was there to help. I didn't find any life-threatening bleeds during my quick trauma exam, but I suspected he had two broken ankles. However, I was also concerned about the compression that might've occurred to his spinal vertebra, a mechanism known as axial loading. I feared his vertebrae might have been forced out of alignment, like the wooden blocks of a Jenga game.

Once I finished my physical exam, I announced my treatment plan: cervical collar and spinal immobilization via the vacuum mattress, IV and pain medications en route to Fresno, and a rendezvous with Sierra Ambulance along the way.

"This sounds like a good plan," Otto replied.

I turned to Noah. "I'll handle medical, and you'll be my litter captain," I said. "I want you to put together an extraction plan."

"Copy," he replied as two other rangers arrived.

We quickly applied a C-collar and moved Otto to the vacuum mattress, and then we took our places at the carrying straps. Since I was closest to the head, it was my duty to call out the moves. In an odd way, I felt as if I were back climbing *Highway Star*, balancing time and tactics, the microcosm and the macrocosm, and the patient care I needed to do *right then* and those interventions that could be performed during the long transport to the hospital. I felt confident knowing that, like on my climb, Noah and the rest of the YOSAR team had my back. They wouldn't let me fall.

"Is anyone not ready?" Noah asked and, when there was no response, said, "OK, lifting on three."

We moved Otto to the vacuum mattress, applied rolled towels to each side of his head to prevent movement, then lifted him to the gurney, and wheeled it toward the ambulance. En route, I started an IV, gave him Fentanyl for pain and Zofran for nausea, and by the time I transferred care to Sierra Ambulance, Otto was pain free and had forgiven Inge for her inattentiveness. "Sorry I said those things," he said, taking her hand. "I was hurting."

Later, as I finished my patient-care report, I looked at my times on the dispatch log and discovered my total on-scene time was eleven minutes. While it wasn't the ten minutes suggested for a critical trauma patient in the Prehospital Trauma Life Support class, it was still good. Otto didn't have life-threatening injuries, so I had thought it was wise to move methodically.

"Slow is smooth," Sam had told me at Yellowstone. "And smooth is fast."

I was proud of my performance and felt like I'd taken a small step toward becoming proficient in search and rescue. Nevertheless, I wondered how I'd perform when the patient was farther up the trail. Would my physical training pay off? Could I reach a patient and run the call effectively under those circumstances?

With the high number of search-and-rescue missions in Yosemite, I knew I'd soon find out.

SOMEBODY'S WORST DAY

"YOU MUST GIVE UP THE LIFE YOU PLANNED in order to have the life that is waiting for you."

I've always loved that quote from one of my favorite writers, Joseph Campbell, but I had never grasped its full significance until one night when I turned on my computer and found an email from a fire department in Los Angeles inviting me to interview for a firefighter position.

I'd taken the written exam months before in a huge pavilion at a fairground in California. The fire department there had apparently been so worried about the possibility of cheating that there were rumors they had the exams flown in by helicopter and delivered to the testing site in a Brinks truck. That day I stood in an endless line in the blistering heat with my ID and "invitation to test" letter, waiting to check in for the exam. Sweat dampened my dress clothes. Local news agencies, reporting live from the scene, plucked random candidates from the crowd and asked, "How does it feel to be one of thousands applying for a fire job?" Members of the fire department drove by in the engine and blasted the air horn for encouragement. My stomach grumbled something about eating a bigger breakfast next time. After I checked in for the exam, I waited in another terribly long line to get a seat at one of the folding tables that seemed to stretch endlessly to the horizon.

The sheer number of candidates had felt downright depressing. The defeatist part of my mind told me to quit right then and there, but I didn't. I honored my hard work and my dream of being a firefighter and told my bladder it would just have to wait, because the bathroom line was too long. (Whoever had picked the testing site had neglected to factor in that three bathrooms for three thousand nervous men and women were not enough.) I regretted that decision, when it became clear that the test moderator was planning to go over all the directions in their absolute entirety. By then, I'd waited over an hour to check in, an hour to be seated, and half an hour to listen to directions, and my bladder was stretching like a balloon about to pop.

Hours later, I left that test feeling my lowest, questioning not only my career choice but my purpose and place in the universe. In fact, I was so distraught that despite my bladder's protests, I bypassed the bathroom on my way out and hurried to my car. I just wanted to get out of there.

When I started my journey with the National Park Service, I was delighted by the opportunity to experience nature, fulfill a dream to work as a park ranger, and become an all-hazards provider able to operate in every environment, under any conditions. However, my ultimate goal was always to return to Los Angeles to work as a firefighter paramedic. That was the future I'd planned for myself, and it even made sense in the context of Joseph Campbell's "heroic journey," which is divided into three parts:

departure, fulfillment, return. In my life's context, I'd departed from the low-paying metaphorical wasteland of working for a private ambulance company in Compton, California, for the new world of the National Park Service. By running calls at Yellowstone and Yosemite, I'd undergone a series of trials—each mounting in difficulty—and had improved as a paramedic and been certified as a firefighter. To complete the journey, I would now return to L.A., strengthened by the tribulations, renewed, and ready to save lives. It was a classic "voyage and return" as seen in *Gladiator*, *The Matrix*, and *Back to the Future*.

There was only one problem: I didn't want to go back.

I had fallen in love with seasons and weather again, felt like I'd discovered my tribe, and loved the challenges of working as a remote medic. There was something about the way steam rose off Yellowstone's Grand Prismatic Hot Spring at dawn or how the sun set over El Capitan in Yosemite, leaving its granite walls glowing like golden molten lava, that made me realize we are made of mountains, with rivers running through our veins. I didn't want to simply visit nature. I wanted to make it my permanent residence.

I took a deep breath, then emailed the fire department and politely replied that I was no longer interested in the Los Angeles position. As I hit send, I knew my decision wasn't rational. I was choosing to continue working seasonally over the possibility of a permanent job in California, but to be honest, I was excited about what the unknown held.

"Follow your heart," Hannah had said to me before she left Yellowstone. At long last, I would.

As I turned off my computer that night, I resolved to research permanent firefighter paramedic jobs in mountain towns in Wyoming, Utah, Colorado, Montana, and Washington State.

It was at about the same time that Roger Graham suddenly began slurring his words while reading a bedtime story to his children.

Ambulance 3, respond to the lodge for a thirty-seven-year-old male with stroke-like symptoms.

"It can't be," I said to Ben as we drove over. "When was the last time you saw anyone under sixty having a stroke?"

"Never," replied Ben. "But let's move fast just in case."

"Copy," I replied, parking the ambulance and calling us on-scene.

Yosemite Valley Lodge was a large wood-and-glass building with 245 rooms and majestic views of Yosemite Falls. It was a favorite among families. As Ben and I pulled out the gurney, we were both expecting the type of call we'd run dozens of times. The family went for a hike, and Dad overexerted himself and didn't drink enough water. Then, since the grandparents were along on the trip and offered to watch the kids after dinner, Mom and Dad went out for drinks on a mini date night, and now he was slightly drunk, dehydrated, and slurring his words. This was not an uncommon scenario, since symptoms of hypoglycemia often mirrored a stroke, and we'd be able to simply tell him to rehydrate with small sips of water or Gatorade and to rest and enjoy the remainder of his time in the park.

But when an elderly woman hurried out to meet the ambulance and said, "Come quick. Room 38! It's my son!" there was something in her trembling voice that told me we'd be dealing with something more unusual and serious.

Luke—my dashing, badass, all-hazards, law-enforcement-ranger roommate—rolled up in his patrol car and jumped out to assist. "Where do you need me?"

"Grab the front of the gurney," I said quickly.

"When did this happen?" Ben asked the woman, following her to the door.

Since Ben was lead provider on this call, I'd help out by taking vital signs and driving to the hospital if necessary

"Ten minutes ago," the woman said. "Roger was reading a bedtime story to the boys, and he just slumped over suddenly."

The grandmother directed us to the room, which looked like a typical family vacation room, with sprawled suitcases, stuffed animals, and special treats. Everything looked normal until we spotted the wife and two boys, aged four and six, crying in the corner. Their father was lying in bed, slumping on his right side with a copy of the children's classic *Goodnight Moon* beside him.

Ben, Luke, and I knew immediately that it was go time.

Roger was a tall man wearing jeans and a golf shirt.

Ben directed me to perform a stroke exam and obtain a set of vital signs, then turned to Luke. "Get a blood sugar."

I quickly introduced myself. "Roger, can you give me a big smile?" I asked, demonstrating a Cheshire Cat grin. Roger was conscious but unable to move his mouth. His lips curved badly to the right, and saliva ran down his chin.

"I have obvious facial droop," I told Ben, before quickly turning back to Roger. "Can you repeat the phrase, 'You can't teach an old dog new tricks'"?

Roger could only whimper.

"Blood sugar normal at 127," Luke announced.

For my last stroke diagnostic test, I asked Roger to straighten both arms out in front of him. "Like this," I said, demonstrating, extending my arms as if I was about to dive into a pool.

Roger extended his left arm into the air but couldn't move his right. He was paralyzed along his whole right side.

"Stroke scale positive in all fields," I announced and grabbed a blood pressure cuff and stethoscope.

I quickly took a set of vitals. As I expected, Roger's blood pressure was elevated and his heart rate rapid.

"We need to get him to a stroke center immediately," Ben said and quickly summoned dispatch. "I'd like to order a life flight helicopter."

Since it was dangerous for a helicopter to navigate the maze of Yosemite Valley at night, we'd meet the bird near the Crane Flats Campground, seventeen miles northwest.

"Launch it," Ben replied. "We'll meet you there!"

It took all three of us to move Roger, as he was unable to help us in any capacity. The copy of *Goodnight Moon* caught in the blankets and fell to the floor as we moved him onto the gurney. His whimpers grew louder as we buckled the seatbelts on the gurney, and tears streamed down his face. Though Roger couldn't speak or move, he knew exactly what was going on, which was why I hated running stroke calls. At least an unconscious patient didn't know what was happening.

As we wheeled Roger to the door, his wife and boys said goodbye. It was absolutely heartbreaking.

Grandma followed us out the door. "I'm coming with you."

"Not sure you can fly," I said. "There's a weight limit for the helicopter—"

"I'm not leaving my boy," she said adamantly. I didn't argue.

We loaded Roger into the ambulance, and Luke jumped in the back to help Ben. I assisted Grandma into the front passenger's seat, hopped into the driver's seat, and sped toward Crane Flats. The road was dark with tiny islands of black ice. Deer appeared like apparitions with antlers, and I swerved to avoid them.

In the back of the ambulance, Ben and Luke started IVs and placed Roger on the cardiac monitor. Meanwhile, in the passenger's seat next to me, Grandma struggled to make sense of the tragedy.

"He was just reading to the boys and all of a sudden—," she managed, her voice trailing off. "Roger's never had any medical problems before."

"I'm really sorry this is happening, but we're doing the best we can," I replied.

Suddenly she turned to me. "I gave Roger some aspirin. That should help, right?"

Aspirin was suggested for chest pain and a suspected heart attack to prevent the clot in the artery from growing. However, you didn't give aspirin for a suspected stroke as you couldn't know for sure if it was caused by a blood clot (ischemic) or a brain bleed (hemorrhagic). If it was a hemorrhagic stroke, giving the patient aspirin—a blood thinner—could potentially make it worse. However, I wasn't about to tell her that; she didn't need that on her conscience. I reaffirmed what was going right with the call.

"Ma'am, you did the right thing by calling 9-1-1," I told her. "We've launched a helicopter, and they'll be taking him to the nearest stroke center."

I could hear Ben and Luke in the back of the ambulance, repeating the stroke exam.

"Can you give us a big smile now?" Luke asked. "Like this? Can you move your mouth at all?" I could tell by their repetitive questioning that Roger's condition hadn't improved.

We arrived at Crane Flats, followed by three law enforcement rangers who would assist with landing the helo. We parked and quickly shut off our lights so as to not interfere with the flight crew's night vision goggles.

Roger continued to make incomprehensible sounds, and tears ran down his face. It sounded like he was trying to say "fuck." That the poor man couldn't even swear correctly felt, in the moment, like the biggest tragedy. A guy having a stroke ought to at least be able to say a big "eff you!" to the universe.

Ten minutes later, we heard the rhythmic sound of rotor blades, and the helicopter descended from the dark. Due to Roger's critical condition, we performed a hot load. As I had suspected, Roger's mother couldn't fly with him due to the weight limit of the chopper, but she thanked us for giving her the extra time with him in the ambulance.

"Goodbye, son," she said as we loaded Roger up. "See you at the hospital."

When the helo departed, Mike and I assisted her into the back of a patrol vehicle, so an LE ranger could take her back to her hotel room and her family who she'd accompany to the hospital. She was stunned and saddened and off-balance as she walked away. The last question I heard her ask the ranger before the car door closed was, "I gave Roger aspirin. That would help, right?"

"I can't say, ma'am," he replied. "But what I do know is he's en route to the hospital now and getting the best care possible."

• • • • • • •

The following day we learned that Roger's stroke had been caused by a patent foramen ovale. A PFO was a hole between the two upper chambers of the heart. This hole was essential for fetal circulation, but for most people, it closed soon after birth. However, if it remained open—or *patent*—a clot could travel from the heart to the brain and cause a stroke.

The diagnosis cast a gray cloud over the otherwise sunny April afternoon. At the medical clinic, we debriefed about the call.

"We couldn't have been faster on-scene," Ben said.

"And the helicopter landed just minutes after we arrived at the LZ," I added.

Luke asked if there was anything we could've done differently.

"Honestly, I don't think so," Ben replied.

"Me neither," I said.

As it turned out, the aspirin Roger's mom had given him had likely helped prevent the clot from getting bigger.

After a moment of silence, I asked a question that had been weighing on my mind. "Did the hospital mention Roger's potential for recovery?"

"Not good," Ben replied, and I didn't ask him to elaborate.

This dedicated father and husband's life was forever changed by a hole in his heart.

Maybe the stroke was the result of a lifestyle choice? Workaholism and stress leading to high blood pressure and artery disease? Perhaps it was a freak accident? Or had it all come down to Swiss cheese?

Hoping for some fresh air, I wandered outside, where I pondered the Swiss-cheese model of accident causation. Dante Orlandella and James T. Reason, professors at the University of Manchester in England, likened human operations and systems to slices of Swiss cheese stacked side-by-side. Risk—the holes in the cheese—was mitigated by different defenses. Therefore, in theory, a lapse in one defense didn't necessarily threaten the entire system, since other barriers could prevent a failure.

"The presence of holes in any one 'slice' does not normally cause a bad outcome," Orlandella and Reason wrote. "Usually, [a bad outcome] can happen only when the holes in many layers momentarily line up to permit a trajectory of accident opportunity—bringing hazards into damaging contact with victims."

My paramedic work had taught me that the Swiss cheese system was built into the human body, with blood vessels contracting and dilating, the heart rate rising and falling, and the pH of the blood balancing between acid and base to achieve the dynamic but balanced state of homeostasis.

Unfortunately in Roger's case, the holes in the Swiss cheese had lined up: the PFO hadn't closed, his condition hadn't been detected by doctors, the process known as fibrinolysis had failed to break down the clot in his blood, and the clot had gone through the PFO and traveled to his brain, all of which created a tragic "trajectory of accident opportunity." And so he'd begun slurring his words while reading *Goodnight Moon*.

Tragedies like this hit me hard, here at a national park. People came here on vacation, happily visiting a magical place like Yosemite or Yellowstone, distanced from the stress and demands of work and daily life, only to experience such an ugly event.

It was a cruel irony for them to undergo tragedy in such a pristine setting.

YOU CAN'T MAKE THIS STUFF UP

AS MARCH ARRIVED, we were dispatched to treat a crazed man with blue hair running naked past the Yosemite Valley Visitor Center. College spring breakers had descended on "nature's grandest temple" and with them law enforcement and EMS calls for drunk kids passed out at El Capitan Meadow, paranoid stoners in the tent cabins in Curry Village, and the aforementioned barefoot jogger, born to run in his birthday suit.

From the visitor center, the streaker ran past the Ansel Adams Gallery, turned right, and dashed toward Village Drive.

"You can't make this stuff up," I said to Sarah, my partner on the ambulance that day, as we arrived on scene and saw the guy cornered by LE rangers in a parking lot near the research library.

It turned out that he was having a bad acid trip. He kept yelling, "YOSEMITE NATIONAL PARK!" at the top of his lungs, sweating, and dancing around, which was scaring families. So we administered five milligrams of the sedative Versed by giving him an intramuscular injection into his right deltoid.

Most of the calls during the spring break window were benign, but when a student from the University of Washington went missing for two days, a massive search-and-rescue mission ensued.

Alex Hulet and his buddies were visiting Yosemite for the first time and had started hiking near Lower Yosemite Falls at 10:00 AM on March 20. From the Lower Yosemite Falls footbridge, they began scrambling over the boulders, but when his friends turned, Alex had disappeared.

"Alex!" they called out.

No response.

"Aleeeeeeeeex!" they tried again. "Come on, man. This isn't funny!"

Nothing.

It was as if Alex had disappeared into thin air or had been the unfortunate victim of some alien abduction.

Alex's friends searched for several hours that afternoon before calling 9-1-1 to report him missing. When he still hadn't turned up the following morning, a BOLO (be on the lookout) was issued, and we ramped up the search.

When you work as a park ranger, there are calls that make you question humanity—like when an idiot left a loaded pistol on a picnic table at Madison Campground in Yellowstone or when gang members tagged trees, rocks, and tent cabins with graffiti in Yosemite. The rescue mission to find Alex that weekend, however, reaffirmed my faith in people.

Park Service employees and volunteers plastered missing person flyers around the valley. California Highway Patrol helicopters flew laps overhead. Canine search teams scoured the boulders and trails at the base of Yosemite Falls, and search-and-rescue teams from Tuolumne County, Mariposa, and Marin County all came to assist YOSAR. These dedicated volunteers took off work and traveled miles to spend hours scouring the woods and searching for a young man they'd never met.

When Alex disappeared, he didn't have his wallet or cell phone on him and was dressed for a short day hike in mild temperatures. His friends had no idea what his direction of travel or itinerary was, but search-and-rescue specialist Arthur Briggs relished such a challenge. From his tiny office in the SAR Cache, Briggs's beautiful MIT-trained mind worked from dawn till dusk, analyzing the terrain, topography, and weather and calculating Alex's potential speed of travel. Like a method actor, Briggs attempted to step into Alex's skin: *Who am I? What do I want? How can I get it? What's in the way?*

The search turned up nothing during the day and was called off late that evening when a weather system pummeled the valley with lightning, thunder, and freezing rain. As I lay awake in bed, listening to the rhythm of rain on the roof, I felt for Alex, out there somewhere. But whether it was illness, injury—or simply being lost—something was preventing him from removing himself from the environment. And now, the rain and cold temperatures meant he was likely hypothermic—or dead.

The next morning, my roommates and I met all the valley law-enforcement rangers and search-and-rescue members at the SAR Cache, and the search ramped up in urgency.

"Alex has been missing for over forty-eight hours in inclement weather," Sarah said at the morning briefing. "We're hoping this will be a rescue, but it could be a recovery."

Sarah began discussing our assignments for the day when suddenly dispatch contacted us on the radio: "All units be advised, a caller believes he's spotted the BOLO in the boulders just off the Valley Loop Trail, a quarter mile east of the Lower Yosemite Falls footbridge."

A family hiking the Valley Loop Trail had recognized Alex, who was barely alive, from the missing person flyers and called it in. We had searched the same area dozens of times, which led us to believe that over the last two days, Alex had been on the move.

Sirens pierced the clear mountain air as rangers sped over to the location in their patrol cars. We followed in the ambulance, trailing yellow-shirted SAR personnel sprinting over to the recovery site. In a strange twist of fate, Alex had been located only a few hundred yards from the SAR Cache.

We pulled up on-scene, grabbed the vacuum mattress, and hurried toward Alex, who was surrounded by SAR personnel. They immediately began holding his head in neutral alignment for spinal precautions.

It was quite surreal to spend days with your eyes peeled for someone on a missing person flyer and then to suddenly see them. The photo used on a flyer like that was often taken on a person's best day, yet we encountered him on his worst. The picture on Alex's flyer showed him in a preppy shirt with short-cropped red hair, and a bright, toothy smile. But when we found him, clinging to life in the mossy boulders, he looked like something from a zombie apocalypse. We'd later learn from the photographs he took before he got lost that he'd likely taken a fifty-foot fall somewhere near Yosemite Point or Sunnyside Bench and had since been on the move, stumbling and crawling through the woods as he sought help.

Alex was drenched and covered with dirt, pine needles, and leaves. It looked as if he scraped up the top layer of earth and formed it into clothes. He was barely conscious, pale, shivering, and his frail body was one big injury. Purple bruises like Halloween paint framed both his eyes and the spots behind his ears. Although we had yet to learn what had happened to him over the last forty-eight hours, the raccoon eyes and other battle signs suggested that Alex had a serious head injury.

Ben was lead for the call and announced his initial treatment plan. "Let's get a cervical collar on him and move him from the rocks to a vacuum mattress."

"Copy," we said, jumping into action.

We quickly applied a cervical collar and moved Alex to the vacuum mattress. We cut away his wet clothes, which clung to his body like dirty Saran Wrap.

As Luke and I performed a rapid physical exam and announced our findings, Ben scribbled notes:

HEAD: Possible skull fracture. 3" full thickness laceration on occipital region. Large avulsion over right eyebrow, puncture wound over left eyebrow.

PELVIS: Swelling and contusions on right hip.

BACK: Multiple abrasions.

EXTREMITIES: 2" full thickness laceration on left leg, bone exposed. Right elbow swelling and contusion. Scattered abrasions.

SKIN SIGNS: Pale, cool, and dry. Wet clothes. Odor of incontinence.

PUPILS: Sluggish, slow to response.

MENTAL STATUS: Altered. Opens his eyes to voice but confused.

TRIAGE CATEGORY: Critical, Trauma Red.

We quickly immobilized Alex on the vacuum mattress and carried him to the waiting ambulance. In accordance with prehospital trauma life support, we were off-scene in less than ten minutes. All of our hours of training and working together had made us a well-oiled EMS machine.

I drove as Ben, Luke, Noah, and Brad Miller, the physician's assistant, tended to Alex in the back of the ambulance. As we raced to Ahwahnee Meadow to rendezvous with a medevac helicopter, I heard them cranking the heat—"We need to warm you up"—starting IVs—"Just a little poke"—and reevaluating Alex's mental status—"What's your name? Where are you right now?"

As we arrived at Ahwahnee Meadow, Yosemite firefighters clad in yellow bunker gear stood by their engines, waiting to help us land the helicopter. As I spotted them—and thought about dispatch, law enforcement, EMS, search and rescue, volunteers, and firefighters—I realized again that it really took a village to save a life in a remote setting.

But as so often happens in rural EMS, there was a problem: "The helicopter needs to turn around due to weather," dispatch said.

"DAMN!" I yelled before keying my mic and assuming a very calm and polite tone for dispatch—and everyone else listening to the radio traffic. "Copy, ma'am. Can we find an LZ outside of the valley?"

The flight team requested Batterson Fire Station, three miles north of the town of Oakhurst. It was an hour and twenty minutes away, but it was our only option.

"We're en route," I replied, spinning the ambulance around and hauling down Southside Drive.

As I drove, veering around impossible corners, I scanned the road for deer and coyotes, but my ears were firmly attuned to the back of the ambulance. I was listening to every word Ben, Luke, Noah, and Brad uttered, and based on their conversation, I could tell when they were seat-belted or standing, starting an IV, or pushing a medication, and I sped up or slowed accordingly. Along with the standard two IVs for a critical trauma patient —warmed saline fluid and anti-nausea medication—they also gave Alex the antibiotic Ancef to prevent infection in his dirty open wounds.

"Alex, open your eyes if you can hear me!" Brad instructed.

"Come on buddy," added Noah. "Open your eyes."

I could tell by their questioning that Alex's mental status was declining fast. But why? I'd assumed his condition would improve with our efforts.

"He's a GCS 7 now," Ben announced.

The Glasgow Coma Scale (GCS) is a neurological scale to rate a person's level of consciousness, based upon their response to a series of basic tests. *Were the patient's eyes open? Could the patient answer basic questions? Did the patient have purposeful movement?* When we first found Alex, he was a GCS 13, meaning he was confused but opened his eyes when we spoke and was able to move his extremities with intention and awareness. But in the ambulance, he wouldn't open his eyes even to a painful pinch and was mumbling incomprehensible words, his extremities lying limply at his sides.

I'd heard about the afterdrop phenomenon with hypothermia, but I'd never encountered such a patient before. According to the literature, the afterdrop phenomenon occurred when a hypothermic patient was rewarmed, and cold blood and lactic acid—a toxin—returned to the heart. As this "bad blood" from the periphery entered central circulation, it could cause a patient's heart rate and blood pressure to drop, known as "rewarming shock," or cause the patient to go into cardiac arrest.

"Alex, can you hear us?" Brad demanded. "Open your eyes!"

"GCS 3 now," Ben said ominously.

A GCS 3 is the lowest the scale goes. That meant Alex was in a deep coma—or dead.

I floored it as Noah brought up the idea of inserting a breathing tube down Alex's windpipe, but Brad said to hold off.

"He still has a gag reflex. He could throw up," Brad said, before calling up to me. "How much farther?"

"Fifteen minutes!" I said.

As we left the park boundary, the road straightened, and my speedometer twitched with speed.

Batterson Fire Station was home to the US Forest Service's Sierra Hotshot Crew, an elite team of wildland firefighters. While the summer season was still a few months away, a few firefighters, dressed in yellow wildland fire shirts and green pants, were standing there to help us land the chopper.

When the flight team arrived, they gave Alex a sedative and paralytic and performed a rapid sequence induction to control his airway by inserting a breathing tube. We quickly moved him into the bird before it lifted off in a whirlpool of dusty wind.

· · · · · · ·

Later, as we drove home, I inquired more about the afterdrop phenomenon. Was the arrival of first responders paradoxically the most dangerous part of the incident? Did the afterdrop phenomenon have a mental aspect?

"Definitely," Brad replied.

Brad explained that a patient in shock would have a fight-or-flight reaction, which increased a patient's respiratory rate, constricted blood vessels, and raised a patient's heart rate to maintain blood pressure and perfusion.

"When first responders arrive, however, it often causes the patient to relax, which can knock out this compensating mechanism, causing the patient's vital signs to crash," he said.

"How do you prevent it?" I asked.

"I always tell the patient that my team is going to help," Brad explained. "But then I tell the patient to keep working with us. Whatever you do, I tell the patient, don't give up now."

Miraculously, Alex survived and returned to the University of Washington to graduate with a degree in cinema and media studies. Soon after, he wrote, shot, and produced a short film about a selfish man who learned to care more for his community, his close friends, and nature in order to win over the girl of his dreams.

21

SWISS CHEESE AND
SILVER LININGS

AS YELLOW MANZANITA BLOSSOMED and California bay flowers bloomed beside sprouting ferns, the summer SAR siters moved into tent cabins. They would live in historic Camp 4 for free during the summer in exchange for assisting with search-and-rescue missions. Late spring arrived in Yosemite Valley, and once again, the end of a seasonal position with the NPS had snuck up on me. Was it denial? Or was something else at work?

As I pondered the months I'd worked for the National Park Service, living in the heart of Yellowstone and Yosemite, I decided that it wasn't denial—it was that living in a national park plunges you entirely into the present moment. Your world simultaneously collapses and expands. It shrinks to your assigned district and yet grows larger due to the full existence you live while there. You live alongside a diverse community of people who value a campfire over a television, conservation over consumption, and shared, spoken stories over social media. You find "a world in a grain of sand" and "a heaven in a wildflower," like the English poet William Blake wrote. And, rather than by a clock, your sense of time is measured by geyser eruptions, the return—or departure—of waterfalls, and the lumbering migration of bison and elk.

I felt like I'd found my tribe with the NPS, and yet I knew my time linking seasonal jobs had to end. At the time, there were no full-time career firefighter paramedic jobs with the agency. I also couldn't become a law-enforcement ranger, since the cutoff age to be hired for a permanent position was thirty-seven, and I was beyond that.

As I took stock of my situation, one could argue I was no better off than when I left Los Angeles to begin this adventure: I still had no permanent job, nor had I saved much money for retirement, and I wasn't any closer to my goal of getting married and having kids one day.

Had it been a mistake to accept that first temporary job in Yellowstone? I didn't think so. I knew I'd changed in ways beyond what might be evident on a résumé. My whole outlook on the world had transformed. I'd become more connected and open, grown as an EMS provider, gotten certified as a firefighter, and learned some basics about search and rescue.

I had just finished applying for a firefighter paramedic job with Jackson Hole Fire/EMS in Wyoming when Erica Cooper, a sixty-seven-year-old woman from Athens, Georgia, took a bad fall way up on the Mist Trail that leads to Vernal Falls.

Sarah radioed me and Luke from the SAR Cache. "Form a hasty team. Get to the patient ASAP and let me know what you have."

"Copy," I replied, quickly changing into my fluorescent yellow NPS search-and-rescue shirt and throwing on my helmet, approach shoes, and black harness. "SAR Grange en route."

The purpose of a hasty team was evident in the name: to reach a victim ASAP. We traveled light and fast. But there was a downside: if the patient was dead or dying, we had minimal gear with which to provide aid.

As Luke and I jogged up the steep paved path, dispatch informed us Erica had fallen on one of the granite steps leading to Vernal Falls, a few miles up the trail. It sounded like a simple ground-level fall, but I never underestimated the Mist Trail. More people had died on that benign-looking path than anywhere else in the park. The reason? Suffering head injuries from slipping on the slick rocks, drowning in the swift current if they fell in the Merced River, or plunging over the waterfalls.

Along with the dangerous trail, I knew Erica's age worked against her. After thirty, our organ systems lost 1 percent of function per year, meaning the body was less able to compensate for shock. With depleted calcium levels, bones broke easier, and simple burns, lacerations, and abrasions caused greater harm, since skin dermis thinned by 20 percent and blood flow to the extremities decreased. Additionally, as brain tissue shrunk, a void was created in the cranial vault, so head injuries could take days to develop and could be more lethal when they did. Plus, given her age, there was also the likelihood that Erica had other issues, such as high blood pressure, irregular heartbeat, or elevated cholesterol. All of this meant I needed to increase my index of suspicion. Vague and nonspecific complaints along with seemingly mild traumatic injuries like a bump on the head or hip fracture could have life-altering effects. As I recalled from my sink-or-swim call at Yellowstone for the woman at the Old Faithful Inn who I found overdosed on narcotics, in shock, and with a massive GI bleed and COPD exacerbation, it wasn't uncommon to be called to an elderly patient with multiple life-threatening conditions occurring all at once. Lastly, we were quickly approaching evening, or "pumpkin time"—as Sarah and the other YOSAR folks called it—when the air ambulance wouldn't be able to land in the valley.

"We need to hurry!" I said to Luke.

"Going as fast as I can!"

In order to work two steps ahead, so as not to fall three steps behind, we requested a carryout team to follow us up with a wheeled litter and technical rescue equipment. By then, "order big and order early" was as much a part of my DNA as my blood type.

"Copy," said Sarah from her command post at the SAR Cache. "Paging out for a SAR litter team now."

Luke and I followed the paved path as it wound up steeply, crossed the Merced River at the 0.8-mile mark, and then continued up and up. Perspiration quickly soaked my bright yellow shirt, leaving large continents of sweat stains. Carrying the BLS bag on my back, I was breathing hard, but I wasn't in the red zone. I knew I could stop at any moment, quickly recover, and still run the call. All the hours I'd spent trail running and working out at the gym were finally paying off: I was now a rescue athlete.

After climbing one thousand feet in a mile and a half, we clamored up the steep steps leading to Vernal Falls. Nature's giant staircase was ripe with dangers and obstacles. The steps were wet from river spray and worn smooth and slick from years of heavy use. Plus, the "stairs" were more like granite blocks. And there were six hundred of them.

Just then, the staircase zigzagged to the right, and we found Erica and her granddaughter seated just below the falls.

I quickly introduced myself and told Erica the worst was over. "My team is going to get you out of here," I said. Remembering

Brad Miller's words of wisdom about the afterdrop phenomenon, I told Erica not to give up. "We're going to get you out, but I need you to keep working with us," I said. "Don't give up now."

Erica winked and flashed a mischievous smile. "Oh, just leave me here to die."

"Grandma!" her granddaughter shrieked, no doubt already familiar with her humor.

Erica was a spirited woman with brown eyes who reminded me of Ruth Gordon in *Harold and Maude*. When I asked if she had any medical problems, Erica told me she suffered from a bad case of "TMBs—too many birthdays."

"Grandma!" her granddaughter said again before turning to me. "I'm so sorry!"

I laughed but knew time was ticking. When I asked about the incident, Erica said she'd tripped, fell forward on her hands and knees, then bumped her head. She hadn't lost consciousness, and her chief complaint was left knee pain, which she rated five out of ten in severity when seated and eight out of ten when walking.

"Would you like something for the pain?" I asked.

"Got any whiskey?"

"Oh my God, Grandma!"

I offered some pain medication, but Erica declined.

Luke finished taking a set of vital signs and informed me that Erica's vital signs were all within normal limits. With more questioning, I quickly ruled out any cardiac, respiratory, or diabetic emergency or an acute traumatic brain injury. I didn't find any visible trauma with my physical exam, so what was left to do was focus on an evacuation plan. Thankfully, Erica didn't have any life-threatening injuries, but getting her down the steep trail would be a challenge. One fall by her, or anyone on the rescue team, could quickly turn critical as night approached.

I informed Erica that we had a rescue team with a wheeled litter coming up the trail.

"I could probably walk down with assistance."

"You sure, Grandma?"

"I think so."

As Erica made a motion to stand, Luke and I quickly helped assist her to her feet. "There," she said. "I can do this."

Erica could bear weight on her knee and didn't feel dizzy, so Luke and I felt comfortable with the current plan. However, we kept the litter team coming up the trail to have a backup plan if anything changed. With a search and rescue, there should always be multiple safeguards in place. "Two is one and one is none," Luke reminded me.

Erica said her knee didn't hurt as much as she thought, but even as we were slow starting down the steps, she winced in pain with each step. If we maintained that pace, Erica would be uncomfortable the entire way and we'd never make it down to the trailhead by nightfall.

"Ma'am, I'd really suggest a litter team," I said.

Erica pondered and finally agreed. I radioed to the litter team to expedite their response.

While her condition wasn't critical, all of the elements of a successful search-and-rescue mission were coming together: Luke and I responding hastily with a litter team following, arriving on-scene and making a good first connection with our patient, and performing a comprehensive patient assessment and evacuation plan.

When the litter team arrived, I assigned Joel as the litter captain. "I'll handle medical, and we'll follow your evacuation plan," I told him.

"Right on, brother," Joel replied. "Let's get this done."

We helped Erica step into a climbing harness and don a climbing helmet, then secured her to a long backboard. Next, we placed the backboard onto the wheeled litter and secured her with multi-directional webbing and straps.

A wheeled litter was basically a stretcher with side railings and a large, thick wheel at the center. Once Erica was secured, we started down the trail with three litter attendants on each side and one scouting the trail ahead of us. Joel walked alongside, overseeing the safety of the entire operation and occasionally switching out SAR team members on the litter to give them a break. "Let the wheel do the work," he commanded.

I walked alongside Erica, checking in frequently about her comfort level and assessing her mental status. I wanted to make sure she didn't have a worsening head injury or delayed brain bleed like we'd seen with the ice skating incident at Curry Village.

As we continued down the trail, slowly navigating over big rocks and through slippery mud sections, I thought about all I'd learned about search and rescue since arriving in Yosemite. I'd participated in over ten SAR missions that winter and had evacuated patients by walking them out, employing crutches, carrying them in a vacuum mattress, or using a wheeled litter.

Now, as we arrived at a steep section of trail, Joel yelled out, "All stop!"

"It's too steep here," he said, looking down the trail with a furrowed brow. "We should set up a technical rescue system here with an anchor and belay line."

I gazed down at the muddy trail. It was the right thing to do. An accident here could prove catastrophic. This section of trail didn't look that steep, but then I remembered the Swiss-cheese model and the importance of having multiple safeguards in place to avoid disaster.

Joel's plan to set up a technical rescue system to lower the litter would delay us. We might not get down before the sun set, but darkness was no longer an issue, since Erica didn't require a helicopter. All of our helmets had headlights, and, best of all, I was working with one of the finest SAR teams in the world.

Like the master rope-rescue technicians they were, Joel and the rest of the YOSAR team assembled a technical rescue system with ropes and pulleys, and we safely navigated the steep section. Once we made it to the bottom of the tricky part, we unclipped the wheeled litter from the rope system and continued on, arriving at the parking lot an hour later.

"How was it, Erica?" I asked as we assisted her out of the harness.

Erica gave me a thumbs-up. "Fun," she replied. "Can we do it again?"

"Grandma!"

I advised Erica to go to the hospital to get an X-ray for her knee and obtain a CT scan of her head.

"I'll go," she consented. "But I'd like my granddaughter to drive me."

I nodded and took her hand. "Thank you, Erica," I said. "I hope you feel better and come back to Yosemite soon."

After Erica and her granddaughter departed, I thanked Joel and the rest of the litter team. They were the true heroes of the call and had performed the most important treatment: extracting Erica from the dangerous environment.

"Our pleasure," said Joel, packing up ropes and rigging devices, readying the gear for their next rescue.

Driving back to Casa de Medicos that evening, as the first stars blinked between the branches of black oak trees, and the moon reflected in the striated, granite mirror of Half Dome, I thought about bringing Erwin Barret back from the dead beneath Lower Yosemite Falls, embarking on the two-day SAR mission that had saved Alex, and taking part in all the other rescues, and I decided there was a silver lining to the Swiss-cheese model.

While the holes sometimes lined up, and a tragedy occurred, there were also many times when, against all odds, a human life was saved. And it was this faith that kept first responders running into burning buildings, starting chest compressions on a failed heart, and dashing up the trail on a search-and-rescue mission.

A few days later, I had just emerged from the medical clinic after a shift when a man hopped out of a white minivan.

"You're Kevin, right?" he ventured.

"Yes, sir," I said.

He looked familiar, but I couldn't quite place him. *Had I run into him at the gym or in a yoga class? Had I encountered him in a local bar? Or had I maybe responded to him on the ambulance one night?*

"I'm Doug," he said. "From the Curry Village ice rink call with Veronica?"

Suddenly it clicked, and I shook his hand warmly.

"How are you?" I said, flashbacks from the call filling my mind. "How is she?" I asked.

Doug pointed behind me. "You can ask her yourself."

"Hi there," Veronica said, stepping out of the van tentatively and handing me a gift basket. "Thank you for saving my life."

Veronica told me that despite her accident occurring over eight weeks ago, she'd needed to use a walker to get around, and I noticed some lingering neurological deficits in her slightly slurred speech and eye movement. "But I'm getting better every day, and the doctor thinks I'll make a full recovery," she said, nodding.

Swiss cheese and silver linings.

Soon we were all hugging and crying, celebrating her courage, the unlikely bond this traumatic event had instilled in each of us, and perhaps, above all else, the tenuous beauty of life.

• • • • • • •

As May arrived, tourists flocked to the valley, and the 9-1-1 call volume increased. I was dispatched to another SAR up the Mist Trail for a thirty-six-year-old woman who'd fainted, and I treated a hiker for heat exhaustion, a man who'd broken his ankle among the rocks of Lower Yosemite Falls, a child who was having an asthma attack at Yosemite Theater, and a concession employee who was suffering from a conversion disorder, a mental condition in which a person experiences unexplained blindness, paralysis, or other symptoms.

On May 4, I responded to the food court at Curry Village once again for a fifty-four-year-old male who'd had a seizure. Our frequent flyer, Leroy.

"Leroy," I said as he woke up, "you should really go to the hospital."

I talked about the importance of getting his blood work checked and his prescriptions updated and the dangers of repetitive head injury syndrome—which can induce dementia-like symptoms long after the injury—but Leroy declined transport.

"I need to go back to work," he said, peering at a few dirty tables.

"Your health is more important," I countered.

"But they need clean tables," he replied, gazing worriedly at families with trays full of food.

I couldn't help but smile. Leroy wasn't just clearing dirty dishes and cleaning tables; he was creating a sacred space for families to dine together, to enjoy Yosemite, and to make memories.

I wanted to thank Leroy for reminding me of the importance of service over self and living for something outside of oneself. I shook his hand and let him know my season in the Sierras was over. "Thank you for all you do!" I told him.

"Come back soon!" he said, cleaning up a circular coffee-cup stain with a blue rag. "I'll be here."

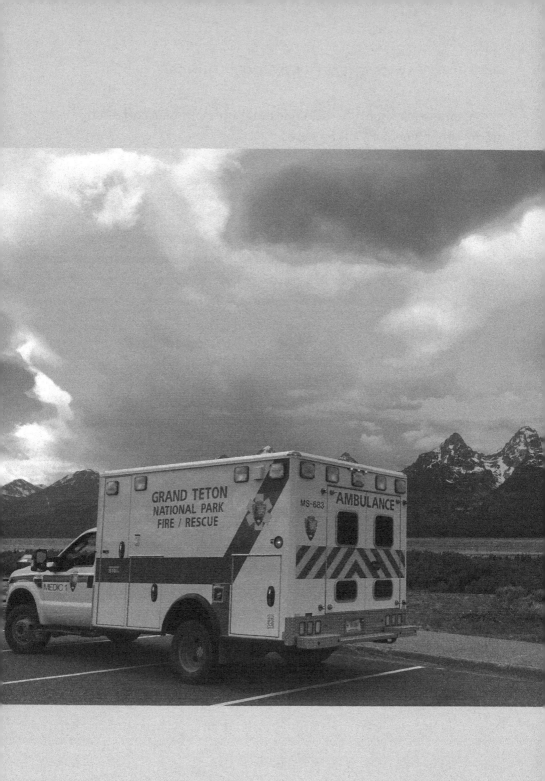

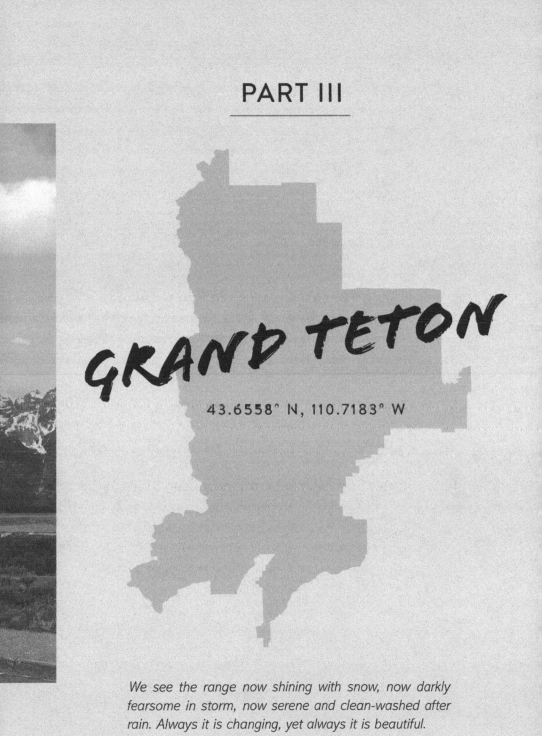

PART III

GRAND TETON

43.6558° N, 110.7183° W

We see the range now shining with snow, now darkly fearsome in storm, now serene and clean-washed after rain. Always it is changing, yet always it is beautiful.

—Fritiof Fryxell, *The Tetons: Interpretations of a Mountain Landscape*

THE WILDLAND-URBAN
INTERFACE

MY PHONE RANG SUDDENLY one afternoon in April 2018. "We need you this summer," the caller said.

The voice belonged to Wes Bradley, Battalion Chief of Fire/EMS at Grand Teton National Park. Like many of the rangers I'd worked with at Yellowstone and Yosemite, Wes was the ultimate all-hazards responder who could operate in all environments, the kind of guy whose email signature was longer than my résumé. As tribute, his staff had once given him a shirt listing all of his certifications on the back: *US Park Ranger, EMS Coordinator, Fire Chief, Fire Officer, Fire Instructor, Apparatus Driver Operator, Firefighter I, Firefighter II, Paramedic, Wildland Firefighter, Pilot, Dive Team Coordinator*, and *Sawyer* (a license to operate a chainsaw and fell trees during a wildland fire incident). Wes was a legendary incident commander—a master of all trades, jack of none—but that afternoon, his voice sounded insistent and urgent.

"Are you interested in working for us as a part-time paramedic?"

I was. Over the past few years, "America's best idea" had become threatened. Big budget cuts had slashed cultural programs, climate-change studies, and scientific research and reduced park staff by nearly two thousand rangers, compromising the ability of the National Park Service to cover basic resource and visitor protection.

Along with this, the United States had dropped out of the Paris Climate Accord. There was an $11.3 billion maintenance backlog. The Endangered Species and Antiquities Act of 1906 was threatened; scientific facts relating to climate change had been removed from government websites; more than a million acres of land had been cut from Bears Ears National Monument in southeastern Utah; and the president wanted the ability to reduce other national monuments without congressional approval. Gone was the optimistic spirit from 2016, when the NPS had celebrated its hundred-year anniversary, and in its place, fear, paranoia, and anxiety had risen up.

But all was not lost.

A resistance group calling itself the Alt National Park Service, composed of over two million people from the NPS, Forest Service, Bureau of Land Management, and other civilian agencies had formed to give voice to the people again. Their mission was to follow the inspiring examples of civil rights leaders such as Dr. Martin Luther King Jr., Cesar Chavez, Harvey Milk, and Jane Addams—the mother of social work—to "stand up for the National Park Service and not let the government destroy our environment and wildlife."

"Sign me up," I replied immediately to Wes, feeling the pulse of patriotism in my veins.

My form of resistance wouldn't be passive but rather active and engaged. I would don the flat hat and green and gray uniform of a park ranger once again to educate people about the NPS mission, the many threats facing our parks, and, of course, hop on the ambulance and save a few lives in the process.

· · · · · · ·

My last night at Yosemite National Park two years earlier had been epic. At Casa de Medicos, Luke, Noah, Ben, Sarah, and Joel threw me a going-away party, complete with a game of pin the tail on "La Grange": beer-drinking participants were blindfolded and spun before attempting to stick a tail on a poster-sized picture of my mug. Law-enforcement and interpretation rangers, entrance gate attendants, and maintenance staff, volunteers, SAR siters, nurses from the medical clinic, wildland firefighters, members of the bear brigade, public information officers, GIS mapping division—old, young, male, female, White, Black, Brown, straight, and gay—they were all there. It was the National Park Service, the heart of America, in all its shining, splendid diversity. The night ended with all of us seated around a campfire, where, as a nod to Sam and Cody at Yellowstone, I threw the cork from the whiskey bottle into the flames, which of course meant we had to down the entire thing.

In the years that followed, I accepted a full-time job with Jackson Hole Fire/EMS in Wyoming, which meant my journey of "rewilding" that I'd begun by moving to Yellowstone was complete. I was back home in the mountains and vowed to never leave again. My full-time job as a firefighter paramedic with Jackson Hole Fire/EMS—an all-hazards agency that, in addition to structure fire and medical emergencies, also responded to hazardous materials incidents, wildland fires, and swift-water rescues—was immensely fulfilling. I was able to buy a home in Jackson through Teton County's affordable housing program, and for the first time in years, I relished having a permanent sense of place, health insurance, and relationships that didn't come with the NPS seasonal employee six-month expiration date.

Despite this, I missed the campfire community of my Park Service family, and on most of the search and rescues in Teton County, I was delegated to stay roadside in the ambulance and wait for a SAR team to deliver the patient to me. I couldn't help but feel that my experience with the NPS was incomplete. I wanted one more shot to integrate all I'd learned at Yellowstone and Yosemite. Was there a park that had high visitation, received the types of medical calls I saw at Yellowstone, and responded to the same high number of traumatic emergencies and search-and-rescue missions as Yosemite? There was. It turned out to be right in my backyard.

Designated as a national park on February 27, 1929, by President Calvin Coolidge and later expanded with the assistance of John D. Rockefeller Jr.—who purchased land to donate in the 1930s—Grand Teton was home to bald eagles, moose, deer, pronghorn, wolves, bears, and bighorn sheep and was comprised of over three hundred thousand acres of rugged mountains, sagebrush meadows, alpine lakes, and the iconic Snake River. Grand Teton fed into Yellowstone via the John D. Rockefeller Jr. Memorial Parkway, which, together with surrounding national forests and refuges and private and tribal land holdings, combined to form the 34,375 square miles of the Greater Yellowstone Ecosystem, one of the largest nearly intact temperate-zone ecosystems on Earth.

Working full-time with Jackson Hole Fire/EMS and part-time as a paramedic in Grand Teton, I'd be operating in what was known as the "wildland-urban interface," that dynamic fringe between remote, rural, and urban elements. Working as a paramedic in one of the largest intact temperate ecosystems on earth would mean ample opportunities to practice wilderness medicine. However, with over three million tourists traveling through the park, along with an airport and the very busy gateway town of Jackson, I could also expect the kind of urban calls I experienced in Los Angeles. My goal for the summer? Let working in Grand Teton be the culmination of all I'd learned thus far about wilderness medicine and being an all-hazards responder.

Like both Yellowstone and Yosemite, Grand Teton had a history of big accidents and emergencies: climbing fatalities, rockfall incidents, wildland fires, drownings, vehicle accidents with tourist buses, and grizzly bear attacks reminiscent of the movie *The Revenant*.

There were also the kind of bizarre incidents that could only occur in a national park.

"Check this picture out," Wes said, as I stopped by headquarters one afternoon to pick up my badge and nameplate. "We're running a cardiac arrest, and there's an elk stuck in a tree in the background."

I leaned in close to look. I hadn't known that elk could get their antlers stuck in tree branches—but evidently, they could. The patient's face and identity was obscured by the rangers providing care, but sure enough, a bull elk stood immediately behind them, its antlers pinned to a spruce tree.

Wes told me about another time a motorcyclist from Minnesota got hit by a pronghorn, an antelope-like animal with curving black horns.

"You mean the biker hit the antelope," I clarified.

Wes shook his head. "No, the car in front of the biker hit the pronghorn, and it catapulted into the air and slammed into the motorcyclist!"

"What are the odds?"

The pronghorn—which also happens to be the second-fastest mammal on earth—had busted up the motorcyclist pretty badly. "Broke both his collarbones, a hip, and fractured his spine."

There had also been a recent grizzly bear mauling. A local hunting guide and his client had killed an elk in the national forest just outside the park and returned the following morning to pack it out. Three grizzlies—a sow and two cubs—charged the pair as they were harvesting the meat. The client survived, but the guide succumbed to his injuries.

Despite its many dangers, Grand Teton was also a place where incredible rescues seemed to occur on a regular basis. It was as if the wrathful energy vortexes here were locked in combat with miraculous recoveries.

On March 3, 2017, a sixty-one-year-old man from Idaho was backcountry skiing in the park when he went into cardiac arrest at ninety-four hundred feet. His family performed CPR, until a local emergency physician, Dr. Will Smith, short-hauled into the scene via a Teton County Search and Rescue helicopter and brought the patient back to life using an AED.

Another time, Dora Davis from Oklahoma started yelling at Rachel LaThorpe for stealing her parking space outside the Jenny Lake Visitor Center one summer day in 2017. Dora got so worked up, screaming and cursing, that her heart stopped. Suffering an out-of-hospital cardiac arrest was usually the end for most people, but it was Dora's lucky day because Rachel—the woman she'd just been cursing at—was a nurse and began CPR. Teton rangers responded and continued treating Dora, and days later she walked out of the hospital with full neurological function.

There was also a freak storm in 2010 during which seventeen people, hunkered down in the rocks beneath the 13,766-foot summit of Grand Teton, had been struck by lightning. While one man fell five hundred feet to his death after being struck, all of the others were rescued and survived.

These were a few of the miraculous tales often told, but equally impressive were the simple day-to-day EMS operations, where AEDs were strategically placed around the park, the majority of the staff was trained in basic CPR and first aid, and EMTs, park medics, and paramedics worked with an expanded scope of practice and progressive treatment protocols that helped save countless lives.

Of course, this little pocket of excellence in the Tetons didn't happen by accident. It resulted from a multiagency response: dispatch, Grand Teton National Park, Jackson Hole Fire/EMS, Teton County Search and Rescue, as well as local and state law enforcement entities. They were all critical players, but it began at the top, with the medical directors who oversaw the programs. At Yellowstone I had the honor of working with Dr. Luanne Freer, the pioneering woman who started Everest ER; At Yosemite, I had the privilege of working with Dr. Ralph Groves; and in the Tetons, I would operate under the inspired direction of Dr. AJ Wheeler and Dr. Will Smith.

Dr. Wheeler grew up in Sugar Grove, Ohio, attended Otterbein University, and went to medical school at the Ohio State University. He was planning on working in sports medicine after graduation but then rotated in the emergency department and loved it. He went on to complete a wilderness-medicine fellowship with the Wilderness Medical Society and earn a Diploma in Mountain Medicine. He now worked as an emergency-room physician at St. John's Medical Center in Jackson and was also the medical director for Grand Teton National Park, Teton County Search and Rescue, and Jackson Hole Fire/EMS. He was an avid outdoorsman and an ultramarathoner. At the EMS refresher, he also gave one of the best lectures I'd ever heard on pain management, especially for rural/remote EMS providers, and taught us how to think of pain control as a "recipe."

"Fentanyl works fast. But it doesn't last long, so your patient's pain level is always dipping and spiking," Dr. Wheeler began. "So on these long transports, we use Fentanyl initially to get the pain controlled and then maybe switch to Dilaudid, which has a longer half-life."

Dr. Wheeler also spoke about other medications at our disposal for pain management, such as Ketamine and Toradol, and really changed the way I thought about pain control. Until then, I'd memorized everything about those medications—their indications, contraindications, side effects, and dose—but he explained further how to effectively use them in an informed, enlightened way.

As for Will Smith, as an MD and a paramedic, he was arguably one of the busiest doctors in America. Along with being an emergency room physician at St. John's, Smith was also the medical codirector for Grand Teton National Park, Teton County Search and Rescue, Bridger-Teton National Forest, and Jackson Hole Fire/EMS. Dr. Smith also served as the medical director for the National Park Service in Washington, DC, and for several other public and private agencies. In addition, he was a clinical faculty member at the University of Washington School of Medicine and a lieutenant colonel in the US Army Reserve. He had completed three deployments in the Middle East, including a stint at Baghdad ER, and several other missions around the globe.

Dr. Wheeler and Dr. Smith were amazing. If they weren't working in the emergency department, they were out responding to SAR missions with Teton County Search and Rescue, often snowmobiling, hiking, helicoptering, or skiing in to reach their patients. Yet despite their impressive résumés, both were super humble and friendly, preferring to be called by their first names, AJ and Will.

Before I worked with Dr. Freer at Yellowstone, Dr. Groves at Yosemite, and Will and AJ in Jackson Hole and Grand Teton, the only contact I'd typically had with my medical directors consisted of seeing their photocopied signatures at the bottom of protocol pages. But these doctors were different: available, active, engaged, and even present on calls. There was nothing like consulting an ER doctor by simply looking over your shoulder and saying, "Hey

Will, are you seeing a heart attack on this EKG?" or "AJ, how about Fentanyl and Ketamine for this patient?"

From Will, AJ, and Wes at the top, the EMS excellence in Grand Teton branched off like multiple IV lines into amazing boots-on-the-ground EMS providers like Jeff Baron, a park medic who'd also worked as a ski patroller and wildland firefighter before joining the NPS, and Adam Moore, who had worked in EMS for over thirty-eight years and had run pretty much every type of call there was. Adam was originally from upstate New York and had a deep baritone voice; everything he said rang with a time-in-the-trenches wisdom. He was the Obi-Wan Kenobi of EMS, at whose feet we prostrated ourselves.

There was also a volunteer, Daniel Simon, nicknamed "Hollywood" because of his love of using moulage makeup for our training scenarios to create bloody patients riddled with stab wounds, bullet holes, or open, sucking chest wounds. Daniel had retired early after earning millions on Wall Street and had donated over forty-six hundred hours as a volunteer.

Hollywood told me he fell in love with being a firefighter and EMT on the very first 9-1-1 call he ran. "There was something about the way the patient shook my hand and said thank you," he explained. "In all my years in the business world, I never received that kind of appreciation."

Sandy Graham was a bubbly, blonde college student who talked how she texted. "For realz," she agreed when I told her that I found working as a national park paramedic more intense than Los Angeles. "OMG! This summer will be perf!" Sandy was interning as an EMT to learn more about emergency medicine. She attended Penn State and dreamed of going to med school one day. As I got to know her, I realized her abbreviated way of talking was more about poking fun at her generation than representing it. Sandy hid a fierce intellect and an iron-will work ethic behind her sunny demeanor.

Another law enforcement ranger had recently arrived in the Tetons after having completed a top-secret mission in an undisclosed location. When he wasn't working seasonally for the NPS as a law enforcement river ranger, he had a different type of all-hazards job: serving as a Green Beret for the Army National Guard.

"Wow, I've never shaken the hand of a special ops soldier before," I remarked to Jeff, the park medic, at the EMS refresher after having met him. "I think he broke a few fingers."

· · · · · · · ·

At Grand Teton, I also had the honor of working with the Jenny Lake Climbing Rangers—the renowned rescue team that had been profiled by CNN and was as accomplished in backcountry searches and helicopter rescue as Yosemite Search and Rescue. They were all elite climbers and mountaineers. Many of the "Jenny Lakers" also worked as LE rangers, including two who, on the afternoon of May 28, put me through a Standardized Field Sobriety Test (SFST).

"Follow the tip of my pen with your eyes without moving your head," a ranger named Brennan commanded, as another one looked on. "Do you understand?"

Prior to working for the NPS, Brennan had served four tours overseas during his five years with the Navy, embedding with the Marines as some kind of top-secret information specialist, then attended Cornell, where he'd won a national championship in wrestling.

"Yes, sir," I replied, feeling uptight and tipsy.

"Let's begin," Brennan said, moving his pen in a vertical line to the right.

I tracked the blue Papermate with my eyes, or so I thought.

"Don't move your head," ordered Brennan. "Focus on the tip of my pen."

"Sorry."

As Brennan's hand reached far right periphery, he held it steady for a few seconds, and the other ranger leaned in close, observing and then scribbling notes.

Brennan then moved his pen to the left. "Keep your chin tucked and arms at your side."

"Copy," I replied, drunkenly.

Luckily, I wouldn't be going to jail that evening. Instead, I was participating in a wet lab, also known as drinking for science. The LE rangers at Grand Teton needed to practice their field sobriety tests to study the subtle physical and mental changes of someone operating a vehicle or boat while under the influence of alcohol. Since the rangers needed people, I—as a proud US citizen who desired to serve his country in any way possible—volunteered to slam a few drinks and participate in the "roadside Olympics."

We volunteers were instructed to arrive at the wet lab with loose fitting clothes and an empty stomach, so we could get "dosed" faster. It was easy to spot someone totally wasted; our goal was to get our blood alcohol content (BAC) to around 0.08, the legal limit, so the LE rangers could learn to spot impaired drivers in that gray area.

The event began with my signing in with two Wyoming Highway Patrol officers, Kenny and Chip, who'd be running the event. They were good ol' Wyoming cowboy cops. Kenny requested my weight, and then Chip consulted an elaborate chart before standing like a bartender and asking, "Whatcha' drinking?"

Bottles of vodka, gin, and whiskey, along with mixers like orange juice, cranberry juice, Coke, and 7 Up resided on the table behind him. Evidently, beer and wine took too long to get someone dosed. The drinks had been donated by the state liquor store, and the plethora of bottles reminded me of one of the parties we'd held at Casa de Medicos in Yosemite.

"Whatcha' drinking?" he asked again.

I couldn't decide. It was stressful ordering drinks from a police officer who was wearing a full duty belt. "Umm. Vodka, please."

"Titos, Absolut, or Ketel One?"

When I decided on Titos, Kenny filled a tall glass and handed it to me. "Your tax dollars hard at work," he said. "You have twenty minutes to finish this."

I added some ice and cranberry juice to the towering drink and then joined the small circle of fellow volunteer drinkers standing in the corner. We were a ragtag group of park employees, buddies, girlfriends, and wives.

"Cheers," I said, raising a glass. "Here's to free drinks. On a Tuesday afternoon. At Grand Teton headquarters!"

Our group was shy and quiet at first, sneaking sips with watchful eyes and hiding our drinks like high schoolers at a family reunion. But as the alcohol kicked in, we grew louder, and the smallest things started to seem really funny. As we hurried to finish our drinks in the twenty-minute timeframe, LE rangers arrived in full uniform, adorned with guns, tasers, pepper spray, and spare magazines.

"Time's up," Kenny announced like a bartender at closing time. "Finish your drinks!"

Chip handed me a plastic straw and ordered me to exhale into a breathalyzer. "Your BAC is 0.11," he whispered, so none of the LE rangers would hear. "You're legally intoxicated."

The first field sobriety test I performed was called the seated battery. Brennan told me this test was perfect for people who couldn't stand and walk the line, such as boaters at Glen Canyon and Lake Mead or folks in wheelchairs.

"Do you see a lot of people in wheelchairs under the influence?" I asked, incredulous.

"You'd be surprised," replied Brennan.

The seated test consisted of following a pen with my eyes, so they could study my nystagmus, the involuntary eye twitching displayed when someone was under the influence of alcohol or a drug like Ketamine. Next, I was asked to close my eyes, lean my head back, and touch the tip of my nose with my forefinger. They also had me perform some tests involving a complex series of hand claps, like playing pat-a-cake, pat-a-cake with myself.

As the afternoon wore on, teams of LE rangers cycled through my station, taking turns practicing their seated battery tests. Every now and then, Chip would wander over to give another breathalyzer.

"You're only a 0.074," he said near the end of the session with a slight tone of disapproval. "Want to get dosed again? I can make you another drink, no problem."

It was quite strange having a cop offering to make me another drink. If I declined, would I be taken to jail for refusing a peace officer? If I consented, could I be arrested for public intoxication?

"I've had enough," I replied, "but thanks anyway."

"No problem," Kenny replied, slapping me on the shoulder. "We really appreciate you coming out to help."

Following the seated battery, I performed the standing SFSTs you normally see at a roadside test—horizontal gaze nystagmus, the heel-to-toe walking, standing on my right leg with the left extended out in front of me while counting, "ONE one thousand, TWO one thousand . . ."

"Keep your arms at your sides," ordered Brennan.

"THREE one thousand, FOUR one thousand . . ."

"Keep watching your raised foot."

"FIVE one thousand," I continued, stumbling over. "SEVEN one thousand . . ."

The evening ended, as drunken nights often did, with a knock on the door and a Dominos delivery guy showing up with pizza.

As we ate, Kenny and Chip discussed the tests and tallied scores for each participant.

"Let's see how Kevin did," Chip said, clicking on an Excel spreadsheet.

"Where we eating breakfast, boys?" I joked, knowing that if this had been a real-life test, I'd be spending the night in the slammer.

Kenny said that five of the six LE ranger teams would've arrested me for driving under the influence. "Which makes sense because he was a 0.04 BAC and below the legal limit when the last team tested him," he concluded. "Nice job, everyone."

I was impressed with the LE rangers' DUI assessment skills, and the wet lab proved valuable for me as well. I realized that I'd gone over the legal limit much faster than I'd have initially suspected, and that I could be arrested for impairment if I were driving erratically even if I was below the legal limit. Most importantly, I discovered I could also use the horizontal nystagmus gaze myself as a test on the ambulance if I had to assess a patient with an altered mental status and wanted to rule out—or in—the presence of alcohol or certain drugs. I could also use some of the seated battery tests if I ever had a patient suffering from high-altitude cerebral edema (HACE), and I wanted to assess the patient's ataxia (unsteady gait) but didn't want to have the patient walk, lest one trips and falls.

The wet lab finished around 9:00 pm, and the LE rangers gave all of us volunteers rides home. Since I lived outside the park in Jackson, Kenny gave me a lift in his Wyoming Highway Patrol vehicle.

"That was cool," I said as I hopped out. "Even the SFSTs were fun! We should do it again some time."

"Let's hope not," Kenny replied, driving off.

· · · · · · ·

Following Memorial Day, all of the LE rangers and seasonal paramedics at Grand Teton had completed their field training, and there was a sense of the summer season revving up. Guests flocked to the park and had a barrage of questions.

When do the deer turn into moose? Do bears poop when they hibernate? Does the scenic float on the Snake River end where it begins?

"No, ma'am," I replied. "It's not a lazy river at a water park."

What does Grand Teton mean?

This question was always difficult to answer, especially when there were young kids around. "Well, sir," I began, "as the French trappers arrived in the area in the 1800s, they must've been quite lonely, because when they saw the mountains for the first time, they didn't have lofty, enlightened thoughts—they decided the jagged peaks looked like big female breasts, hence the name, Grand Tetons."

Along with these questions, calls came in for animal traffic jams with bison or bears, for a woman wearing a pink leotard who let her dog off leash on the Taggart Lake Trail—in this case, a pug wearing a white coat—for cars running past the Moose and Moran Entrance Stations without paying, and for one lady who dialed 9-1-1 multiple times because she needed assistance securing a canoe to the top of her Mercedes. I also caught a BOLO for a motorist who'd driven away from a gas station with the nozzle and half the hose sticking out of his minivan. Another night, when a motorist fled on foot after a traffic stop, the Colter Bay law enforcement rangers chased him into the woods, only to suddenly spot a grizzly bear in the green glow of their night vision goggles.

"We stopped pursuing the suspect because the scene was no longer safe," the ranger explained.

Fortunately, the suspect wasn't eaten, and the rangers arrested him the following day at a nearby ranch.

Despite Teton's impressive rescue record, the summer started off with some grim fatalities. During a scenic float on the Snake River, a rafting guide was swept under a log jam and drowned, and just south of Yellowstone, an RV rolled and crushed a thirteen-year-old boy to death.

But fortunately, we saved a few lives too. One afternoon in late May, I was parked in a lot at Jackson Hole Mountain Resort to receive a skier with two badly broken legs. Kip, twenty-two, was on a backcountry ski trip with his buddies and had been traversing a ridge when he slipped and slid a thousand feet down into some rocks, snapping both legs like chicken bones.

An off-duty ski patroller reached Kip first, then Dr. AJ Wheeler inserted near the scene in a Teton County Search and Rescue helicopter and skied down to help the patient. Since the pilot on the helo that day wasn't certified to perform a short-haul rescue, the Jenny Lake Rangers were requested to respond from Grand Teton. They arrived in the park's helicopter and extracted Kip via a hoist rescue, then flew the patient to me. I was on-shift with Jackson Hole Fire/EMS that day and assigned to the ambulance.

Chris Ainge was the Jenny Laker performing the short-haul rescue that afternoon. He'd been a climbing ranger for over twenty years and had helped save dozens of lives. I was aware he'd recently reached the mandatory LE ranger retirement age of fifty-seven and would be retiring shortly. I wondered if this would be the last time he'd dangle beneath a helicopter and receive a bird's-eye view of the Tetons. Like an astronaut, would he miss floating in space and admiring the curve of the earth, up in that celestial space?

Whether or not it was bittersweet for him, Chris was all business when he landed safely with the patient and gave me a hand-off report. "Possible bilateral tib/fib fracture of both lower legs," he said. "Dr. Wheeler gave him Ketamine on-scene."

As Chris gave me the patient hand-off report, I made a point of thanking him for his amazing work on this rescue, and on all the others.

Our patient, Kip, was a snow bro who lived and worked at a slopeside hostel and repeated words like *gnar gnar* and *pow pow* when he spoke. As we drove toward the hospital, I performed the nystagmus gaze test and confirmed that the Ketamine was still in his system. I knew it by the involuntary twitching of his eyes I'd learned about during the wet lab—and by Kip's request for an additional treatment: "Please," he pleaded as we passed an Albertson's grocery store. "I just need peanut M&Ms."

I told Kip he had two badly broken legs and possibly some internal injuries, and we couldn't stop.

"Aww come on, bro," he pleaded with heavy-lidded eyes. "Some peanut M&Ms!"

· · · · · · ·

The first critical call I ran came when I was dispatched to a twenty six-year-old woman named Abby, found seizing on the bike path near Windy Point, south of Taggart Lake.

As I arrived on-scene, I spotted her bloody, scraped helmet and twisted bike, suggesting a high-impact accident.

"Did she hit her head and then have a seizure? Or did she have a seizure while she was riding and then crash?" I asked an Australian couple who'd stopped to help and covered her with some jackets.

"I dunno," the man replied. "We just found her here."

"Is she alone?"

"Yeah, mate."

Abby wore typical road biker gear, and her arms were covered with abrasions. Her head was bleeding badly. The Australian couple had called 9-1-1, covered her with a windbreaker and fleece, and had placed a towel under the open wound in her head. The towel was dirty, however, and probably wasn't helping.

Though we weren't that far from the town of Jackson, I treated the call like the search and rescue beneath Lower Yosemite Falls because it was a cold and overcast afternoon, and Abby had been lying there a while. We needed to operate fast and get her moving to the hospital, so I only brought a cervical collar and vacuum mattress from the ambulance.

Time and tactics, I thought as I performed a rapid physical exam. *Should I order a helicopter, which would arrive in twenty minutes from nearby Driggs, Idaho? Or would it be better to package Abby and transport her to St. John's Medical Center, about a half hour away? Wait for the helicopter or transport her to the closest hospital that could provide basic trauma care?*

"Always be moving toward definitive care," Dr. Freer had advised me at Yellowstone.

I quickly decided on a ground transport. "Cervical collar, vacuum mattress on-scene," I said to Jeff. "Vital signs and advanced life support en route to the hospital."

Abby was my first big call that summer, and I wanted to get it right. Our first treatment would be to get Abby out of the cool, windy environment and into the back of the warm ambulance. And then, since we had a "short" thirty-minute transport to the hospital, I'd perform all other interventions en route—warming measures, vital signs, an IV, Zofran for nausea, and if she seized again, Versed to control the convulsion.

Our execution was solid. We were off-scene in minutes. As we warmed her, Abby became alert and oriented, so I didn't expect a worsening head injury or brain bleed. We dropped her off at the hospital, and I felt the confidence I'd found in Yellowstone and Yosemite returning. It was great to be back in the green and gray uniform of the National Park Service.

GOOD MEDICINE IN BAD PLACES

MY FIRST TACTICAL EMS CALL in the Tetons came on a Wednesday afternoon at the Flat Creek Inn, just across from the National Elk Refuge, when a man called 9-1-1 saying he was armed, barricaded, suicidal, and wanting to hurt others. Law enforcement officers from the Jackson Police Department, Teton County Sheriff, Wyoming Highway Patrol, and Grand Teton National Park all raced to the scene. I arrived with my crew in the ambulance fifteen minutes later, wearing our bullet-proof vests. By then the hotel had been evacuated and the parking lot blocked off, and the police were all in position with rifles.

We staged the ambulance at a gas station beside the inn, far enough to be out of the immediate hot zone—that area where bullets might fly—but close enough that we could arrive in seconds if anyone got shot.

A two-hour standoff ensued, and when phone negotiations failed, the police stormed the hotel room to find it . . . empty.

The whole episode had been a swatting hoax that some deranged individual had thought was funny. He'd called in a false emergency and then watched it play out in real time on a webcam. They traced this particular caller to Florida.

It was a dangerous and infuriating prank, but I realized I had to be better prepared. Sadly, as active shooter incidents continued to occur with more frequency, it became clear to me that mass violence could happen anywhere, regardless of population size, community structure, or geographic area. Plus, I knew our national parks were a target.

Wallace Stegner, the late, great writer and conservationist, said "National parks are the best idea we ever had. Absolutely American, absolutely democratic, they reflect us at our best rather than our worst." I knew that terrorists loved nothing more than to create fear, hit vulnerable areas, and wound our national psyche.

In rural areas like remote Wyoming, I knew the stakes would be even higher if an incident ever did occur, since getting patients to definitive care within the golden hour wasn't always feasible. The remote location placed extra importance on being able to access and treat patients during those first critical minutes following a traumatic injury. Due to this, and at Dr. Will Smith's suggestion, I enrolled in the Park Service's Counter Narcotics and Terrorism Operational Medical Support (CONTOMS) course and paid my own way.

This one-week, fifty-six-hour tactical EMS class would train me to insert with—and provide medical support for—SWAT and special operations law enforcement teams. The goal was to bring prehospital emergency care closer to the point of injury and provide good medicine in bad places during tactical situations. This meant active shooter incidents, the serving of high-risk warrants, encounters with barricaded suspects, riots, hazardous material spills, emergency ordinance disposals, or other mass casualty terrorism incidents. While some people didn't feel EMTs and paramedics should enter such dangerous situations and instead ought to wait far away in the cold zone, my classmates and I were comfortable with the personal risk if it gave us the chance to save a lot more lives.

The course was held in June at the Center for Tactical Medicine in Alexandria, Virginia and was facilitated by the US Department of Health & Human Services and US Park Police. The fifty students in my class were from state and federal agencies such as the National Park Service, US Park Police, US Navy, Immigration and Customs Enforcement, the Department of Homeland Security, and SWAT teams from around the country. Some students were EMTs, others were paramedics, and a few were physicians.

The majority of students were attached to SWAT teams that operated in hot zones with direct threats like active shooters. At Grand Teton, however, we followed the Rescue Task Force (RTF) model. With the RTF concept, after initial law enforcement entry had isolated the threat, a combined EMS and law enforcement team could enter the warm zone—an area that's been cleared by the police but may not be secure—and begin patient care. Along with operating in the warm zone to provide indirect threat care, the RTF program also emphasized creating a casualty collection point, a location used for assembly, triage, medical stabilization, and subsequent evacuation of casualties.

During class, we logged long twelve-hour days of lectures, ballistics labs, and tactical scenarios in the early-summer Virginia heat. We practiced tactical movement and clearing rooms, searching OPFOR (opposing forces) for weapons and handcuffing them, performing emergency surgical airways, applying tourniquets, and relieving a collapsed lung with a chest dart, as well as learning patient drags, lifts, and carries.

My tactical kit for the CONTOMS class consisted of a bulletproof vest, ballistics helmet, safety glasses, tactical assault gloves, an individual first-aid kit—stocked with tourniquets, bandages, decompression needles, occlusive dressings and hemostatic agents—and an orange rubber training pistol that I was to protect and keep on my person at all times. But as I followed Mateo, my instructor, down a long hallway for a sensory deprived assessment scenario, he handed me a blindfold.

"Wear this," he said, placing it over my eyes, "and don't remove it until the scenario is over."

The purpose of the sensory deprivation patient assessment skill was to test my ability to locate a wounded police officer in a large room under blackout conditions, assess his injuries, and provide lifesaving treatment, all while never lifting any part of my body more than eighteen inches off the floor or giving a noise or light signature that would allow the OPFOR an opportunity to shoot me. Having a skill like this was important, since people rarely got shot in clean, well-lit, and secure surroundings. If someone needed help, we needed to reach them anytime, anywhere, and under any conditions.

"Questions?" asked Mateo. He was a SWAT Team member with the US Park Police. He was a man of few words and had a "hard to kill" look like the bald, muscle-bound mob boss at the end of a video game.

"No sir," I said, adjusting my blindfold to get rid of a sliver of light.

Mateo stopped at the doorway to a large room. "What's the color of blood in the dark?" he asked rhetorically. "Wet! . . . You can begin."

"Copy, sir!"

Now blind, I dropped to my knees, then eased myself onto my stomach and started scuttling forward, sweeping my arms and legs in wide circles, searching for my patient.

"Rescue!" I yelled, letting the injured officer—or anyone else—know I was there to help.

I could hear faint moaning from an injured person coming from somewhere in the distance, and I sped up.

"Keep your butt down!" Mateo yelled. "Stay low!"

I found my way to the wall and could now perform a right-handed search. I'd learned this technique at the National Park Service's Fire Academy, and it was the best way to clear a room in low-visibility conditions. I would first follow the wall around all four corners as I searched for the wounded officer before attempting to locate him in the center of the room.

"Hurry!" Mateo hollered. "Your brother in blue is dying."

"Rescue!" I said again, slithering forward and making snow-angel shapes with my body as I searched. "What's your location?"

"Stay low," Mateo yelled. "Bullets were flying here a moment ago."

Suddenly, my sweeping arm contacted a human leg. "Rescue!" I said, positioning myself on the distant side of the victim for cover and concealment.

My patient was a hulking guy who was barely responsive and breathing in fast, shallow clips. Compensated shock, I thought, as I immediately checked his beltline and hands for weapons.

"Stay down!" Mateo roared.

Since I was in an active shooter, tactical situation, I wouldn't use the typical Airway-Breathing-Circulation (ABC) order of assessment and treatment. Instead, I'd use xABC, the x standing for eXsanguination (profuse bleeding). I would need to find and treat that first since mass hemorrhaging was the most likely cause of traumatic death under the circumstances.

"I feel something wet," I announced as I swept the officer's left leg, "So I'm going to immediately apply a tourniquet."

"Tourniquet applied," Mateo replied. "Continue."

I didn't discover any other obvious bleeds, so I checked the cop's airway and breathing by placing my ear near his mouth on the side of his chest to listen for any gurgling.

"Stay low!"

From there, I quickly checked the officer's pulse, which clued me in to his heart rate and blood pressure, then swept my hands over his head, neck, chest, abdomen, extremities, and back. As I did, I heard a weapon hit the floor.

"Gun!" I yelled, sliding the weapon across the room and out of reach.

As I continued my assessment, I could hear my patient's respiratory rate speed up before growing irregular, slowing, and stopping. Had I missed something in my assessment?

"My patient has stopped breathing," I announced. "So I'm going to check for a pulse."

Mateo said my patient no longer had a pulse, and we could stop the scenario. "Decent work," he concluded. "You can remove the blindfold."

Mateo had liked my search technique and movement through the room but said my assessment was hurried and incomplete. "You found the femoral bleed on his leg," he said. "But you missed the sucking chest wound."

"He had a collapsed lung," I replied. "That explains why he stopped breathing."

Mateo added that I shouldn't have thrown the gun across the room. "Any unsecured gun is a threat to you and your entire team." Instead, I should've "safed" the weapon by discharging the clip or kept it on me.

"Yes, sir," I replied, the acid reflux of regret rising in my stomach. "It'll never happen again."

Mateo said not to worry. "Just don't let it happen at the Field Training Exercise at the end of the week."

The course culminated in a written exam on Thursday and an all-day Field Training Exercise (FTX) that lasted well into the night. The FTX was held at a sprawling abandoned building in the woods that looked like some kind of CIA black site. The morning consisted of five one-hour exercises. The first scenario was medicine across the barricade, in which a thief had taken hostages in a bank and had inadvertently shot one in the arm.

"Medic up!" the police officer hollered into the cell phone he was using for negotiation. The hostage taker was on the other end, speaking into a throw phone we'd tossed to him.

My teammate, Andrew—a Navy corpsman—hustled over.

"The guy inside says he'll only talk to a medic," the police officer said, handing Andrew the phone.

"Hello?" Andrew said.

"Who the fuck is this?" the assailant, a role-playing Marine, hissed.

Andrew introduced himself. "I'm a paramedic, and I need you to put a tourniquet on that woman's arm."

"I don't have a damn tourniquet!"

"OK, do you have a belt you can wrap tightly over the woman's arm?" Andrew offered. "Please! You can save a life here."

"Yeah," the man replied. "I can do that."

In our second scenario, a dignitary was shot during a motorcade, and we had to stack up with guns drawn as a SWAT team and move tactically to the vehicle to get him out.

"Rescue!" I yelled as I led our team into a dimly lit room in our third scenario and saw a victim who'd been hit. "Let me see your hands now!"

"I've been shot!" the guy yelled.

"Where's the shooter?"

"He ran out the door," the man managed, struggling to breathe.

"Can you walk to us?" I asked, my training gun still drawn.

"No," the man replied. "I got shot in the leg."

I directed my team to perform overwatch as another medic and I raced toward the patient, quickly applying a tourniquet, then carried him out.

Our fourth scenario had us kicking down a door to simulate serving a high-risk warrant, only to have our teammates get shot by an assailant.

"Shots fired," I yelled, dragging Andrew out of the room to get him off "the X," the spot where bullets were flying. "I've got an officer down," I yelled, reaching into my Individual First Aid Kit for a chest seal to place over his open chest wound.

During the last scenario, we had to enter a room filled with pepper spray and tear gas and remove our gas masks for fifteen seconds. The purpose of this was to show that, despite being extremely uncomfortable, the pepper spray and tear gas wouldn't kill us. Therefore, if necessary, we knew it was possible to enter such an environment unprotected to rescue someone who'd been shot.

As I tore off my gas mask, my eyes immediately started tearing up, and my lungs burned.

Mateo, clad in his gas mask, asked me to state my name, the year, and what class I was taking.

I answered correctly, coughing.

"OK, you can put your mask back on."

I did as instructed, taking a series of deep breaths to wash out the tear gas and pepper spray.

We had to wait for night to fall for the grand finale, a massive training scenario in "the kill house." My teammate, Trevor—a

SWAT medic out of St. Louis—said the rules of the kill house were simple: Nobody was coming to save you. Everything was your responsibility. Kill who needed to be killed. Save who needed to be saved. And always be working.

"Copy," I replied, tightening my grip on my training assault rifle. As the scenario began, I followed Trevor through the "fatal funnel" of a doorway and then, as he swept left, I went right.

Without going into any specific and graphic details that could ruin the experience for the next generation of students who take the CONTOMS class, I'll simply say the final training exercise was a real-time tactical situation involving flash-bang grenades, smoke machines, blackout conditions, speakers blasting siren sounds, and fifty Marines who'd volunteered to act as patients.

My team and I had to locate and treat patients in a hot zone, where we could get shot at any moment. We had to negotiate with hostage takers, apply tourniquets, perform surgical airways, decontaminate hazardous material, pack wounds, and treat collapsed lungs on patients whose lives hung in a delicate balance. We then had to extricate the patients to a casualty collection point outside the building, where they'd be assessed again and routed to the hospital. In short, CONTOMS was the most intense training experience of my life. But it was all worth it the following day, when we had our graduation ceremony at the US Park Police Anacostia Station in Washington, DC. I was so honored to have trained with my classmates that week and stand alongside them that day.

Now I'd be better prepared for the real thing if, God forbid, an active shooter or tactical situation ever happened in Grand Teton or Jackson.

I was ready.

24

GONE TOO SOON

WE COULD'VE BEEN FRIENDS.

I could tell by her climbing shoes in the front passenger footwell of her 2005 Chevrolet Cobalt and the worn copy of Edward Abbey's *Desert Solitaire*. From her headlamp and thirty-two-ounce, wide-mouth, BPA-free water bottle, decorated with National Park stickers, which showed her love of the outdoors and hinted at night hikes through silent forests, to the Wilderness First Responder card in her wallet that proved she cared for others.

We could've been friends, but I was too late. An hour prior to my arrival, Samantha Kennedy, a thirty-seven-year-old woman from Iowa, had parked at a pullout facing the distant 13,776-foot summit of the Grand Teton, brought a 380-caliber handgun to her right temple, and pulled the trigger.

Bang.

There was another type of traveler who visited our Federal lands for the beauty, solitude, and quiet. Unlike the bucket listers in their twilight years who came here to live out their last years in stages of acceptance, some—like Samantha—were the tragic souls whose lives had been interrupted. The suicides.

I first learned about this sad phenomenon at Yellowstone when a concession employee hung himself beside the shadowy banks of the Madison River. And then, a few months later, when a twenty-eight-year-old woman from Ohio named Tracy showed up at the Old Faithful Ranger Station one night after swallowing a bunch of pills. When I asked if she'd ever attempted suicide before, Tracy told me, "Four times by pills and once by car." That night she'd overdosed herself on a medication prescribed to treat hypertension. In high doses, this beta blocker could drop her blood pressure and heart rate precipitously, leading to cardiac arrest. A helicopter evacuation wasn't available due to weather, so we started two IVs, administered a medication called glucagon to combat the effects, and drove her to Idaho Falls. I spent every minute of the three-hour trip with my eyes glued to the woman and the cardiac monitor, praying she didn't die.

I'd hoped those two suicidal subjects were outliers, but I learned that people threatened, attempted, and committed suicide quite regularly in national parks and other federal lands. Since 2002, more than forty people have committed suicide in Grand Canyon National Park alone. The 469 miles of the scenic Blue Ridge Parkway between North Carolina and Virginia is another popular spot, and a rock outcropping in Yosemite is ominously referred to as the "Diving Board." Golden Gate National Recreation Area holds a bleak record: since 1930, over 1,700 people have committed suicide by jumping off the bridge.

It had been dusk when Backcountry Bill and another ranger found the boy hanging from a tree beside the Madison River at

Yellowstone. From a distance, it appeared to Backcountry Bill that the missing boy was simply standing at the water's edge, admiring the rippling sunlight on the watery surface, until he walked closer and saw the rope around his neck. Due to the late hour, Zach and the other Old Faithful LE rangers couldn't cut the boy down. An investigation needed to be performed first, and while all the signs (recent despondent text messages to the boy's friends and a history of major depression) suggested suicide, the LE rangers needed to make sure no foul play was involved.

"We can't cut him down," the ranger in charge of the investigation said, "but we can't leave him out here alone tonight either." There were opportunistic eaters in Yellowstone—bears, wolves, and mountain lions that didn't discriminate—so Zach and another ranger had to watch over the hanging body all night with guns locked and loaded in case a grizzly charged.

After I heard this story, I wondered how that experience affected Zach. *Would hiking through the woods at Yellowstone ever be the same for him? Would Zion's Keyhole Canyon ever radiate with the same celestial white light for the rangers who recovered the bodies of the seven people killed by a flash flood?*

Or how about another ranger friend who responded to a call for a woman who fell overboard at Lake Mead? He dove in without a wetsuit or scuba tank to rescue her. It was only after he swam her up to the boat that he discovered the anchor intentionally attached to her ankles and realized it was suicide. My buddy loved sailing, snorkeling, and scuba diving, but would the experience of being underwater ever be the same for him? And what should he tell his children the next time he was swimming with them and surfaced, and they said, "What's wrong Daddy? You look like you've just seen a ghost"?

Along with all the other demands of the job, park rangers also sacrificed a sense of place. World heritage sites, scenic trails, and majestic turnouts became accident scenes and body recovery sites.

• • • • • • •

Hunched forward over the steering wheel of her Chevrolet Cobalt that was parked facing the Grand Teton, with her blonde hair covering her face, her arms hanging limply at her sides, and a puddle of congealed blood pooling in her lap, it was obvious that Samantha was deceased upon our arrival. But as the lead paramedic on the call, I still had to prove that she was dead beyond a reasonable doubt. I didn't want to be like a medic I knew in California who'd glanced briefly at a guy who'd been shot multiple times, told police officers he was a "dead on arrival," then cleared the scene—only to have the cops call him back a minute later, saying, "Get back here! He's still moving."

To determine death, I assigned my partners the tasks of shining a penlight in Samantha's eyes to ensure her pupils were fixed and dilated and listening with a stethoscope to make sure she wasn't breathing and had no heart tones. My job would be to ensure Samantha had no pulse and to apply electrodes to her four extremities, confirming she had a flatline, or asystole, in multiple EKG leads.

I wanted my interaction with Samantha to be quick and clinical. *Get in and get out.* But I couldn't apply the EKG leads without sitting in the passenger seat next to her, and that's when the call became personal for me. That's when I spotted the climbing shoes, the copy of *Desert Solitaire*. Samantha was no longer the thin, green flatline on the cardiac monitor; she was a fellow climber, backpacker, and first responder. She was one of us.

Your mind goes to strange places when you're seated next to a fellow outdoor enthusiast with an entry wound in the right side of her head and an exit on the left. In my case, I wished Samantha was alive, and we were somewhere—anywhere!—but parked in that dusty pullout overlooking the Teton range.

Maybe I could've introduced Samantha to one of my favorite national parks, North Cascades in Washington. Most people just drive through the park via State Route 20, which follows the Skagit River on the valley floor, and think, "North Cascades is OK." But the moment you leave your car and hike, a mountain wonderland opens up, and you have miles of old growth forests, subalpine meadows, and glaciated peaks entirely to yourself.

With Samantha, I dreamed we could've hiked up to the fire lookouts atop Sourdough, Crater Mountain, and Desolation Peak, where beatnik writers Gary Snyder, Philip Whalen, and Jack Kerouac spent summers in the 1950s, scouting the surrounding forests for blazes and practicing an open-eyed meditation technique that Snyder termed "the art of mountain watching."

Everything you're feeling right now will pass just like clouds across Hozomeen, I could've said to Samantha, pointing at the 8,071-foot mountain with two summits near Desolation Peak. *We can get you help; you'll get through this!*

"Pupils fixed and dilated," my partner said, breaking my reverie. "Not breathing and no heart tones."

I glanced at the cardiac monitor to assess the EKG rhythm in Lead II.

Flatline.

I switched to Lead III.

Flatline.

"Asystole in multiple leads," I told the police officers on scene and printed the EKG strip for my patient care report. I then stepped out of Samantha's Chevy Cobalt and called the on-duty doctor at St. John's in Jackson. "Transcranial, self-inflicted gun-shot wound," I said before relaying the rest of our findings.

"We're good to call it," the doctor replied. "Official time of death is 11:22 AM."

I grabbed the cardiac monitor from the front seat, and we handed the scene over to law enforcement. They would continue their investigation and stay with Samantha until the coroner arrived.

At the ambulance, white disinfectant wipes turned varying shades of crimson as we cleaned the cardiac monitor, stethoscope, and penlight and returned them to the ambulance.

Our EMS universe was back in order. As we drove away, we radioed dispatch that we were clear and available for another call.

"Copy," the dispatcher replied. "Clear and available at 11:45 AM."

With that, the suicide call was completed. But I'd soon discover it wasn't over.

MY DARKEST HOUR

IN THE WEEKS FOLLOWING SAMANTHA'S SUICIDE, I awoke with violent nightmares. Anxious episodes and intrusive flashbacks—along with feelings of grief—rose and fell, suddenly, like thunderstorms over the sagebrush flats. And every time I passed a pullout or a parked car that resembled Samantha's Chevrolet Cobalt, my heart raced, I felt my blood pressure rise, and sweat dotted my forehead.

As I wrestled with the turbulent feelings, I began to feel that everything about being a first responder was immediately dangerous to life and health: the continuous calls, the missed meals, the back injuries from lifting heavy patients, the constant exposure to infectious diseases, the combative patients, and the dreaded night shifts. Even if you didn't get a call, you laid in bed like a coiled spring with one eye open, waiting for the alarm to sound. And when the tones dropped, sudden and shrill, they were like a cattle-prod jolt to the heart. But the posttraumatic stress was far worse than any of these physical factors.

There had been a few specific incidents weighing on me that Samantha's suicide call had brought back up into my consciousness. The first was the case of the missing leg. I'd responded to a motorcycle crash on the highway alongside the Snake River. Joseph Tomlin, a forty-year-old man from North Dakota, had been riding his Harley with his wife, Lucy, on the back when he passed the cars in front of him on a blind curve at a high rate of speed. Neither Joe nor Lucy were wearing helmets.

A Teton County sheriff with years of experience was first on-scene. "Oh God, it's bad," was all he could manage to say.

Joseph and Lucy had smashed into a Suburban pulling a cargo trailer. Lucy was pale and lifeless when we found her, lying prone at an odd, contorted angle in the northbound lane. Her left leg was missing. She'd either died when the motorcycle hit the Suburban, or when she was thrown and collided with a pickup truck.

But where was her left leg?

As we worked to save the life of her husband, Joseph, the police searched for her missing extremity, walking through the surrounding woods and crouching to peer under cars as if it were a family pet that had run off.

Meanwhile, Joseph was in shock and on the verge of traumatic cardiac arrest. As we ventilated him with a bag valve mask, he lay unresponsive on the pavement, missing whole chunks of tissue from his arms and legs. We applied multiple tourniquets and moved him with a backboard into the ambulance, where, with Dr. Will Smith's assistance, we started IVs, inserted a breathing tube, gave him a saline bolus to raise his fading blood pressure, and pushed medication to prevent the breakdown of clots. Ten minutes later, we landed a helicopter on the highway to take Joseph to Idaho Falls. From there he was transferred to University of Utah

Hospital, where he died on the CT scan table, orphaning his and Lucy's two young children.

And Lucy's leg?

The driver of the pickup eventually found it in the back of the pickup bed, lying amidst the haybales. Lucy's body was covered with a green tarp by then, so he simply placed it beside her, out in the open.

It looks like a training prop, I thought, walking back to the ambulance. *Except mannequins never wear shoes.*

Another traumatic experience occurred during a ride I took in the back of the ambulance through Grand Teton with Phil, a sixty-five-year-old stockbroker from San Francisco. It was March, and an hour before we met, Phil had launched his snowmobile into a deep ravine. In such a situation, did you ditch the sled? Or did you hold on tight and try to ride it out? Unfortunately, the Polaris snowmobile user's manual didn't answer such questions. Phil held on and, when he landed, everything broke.

The crash occurred in the Bridger-Teton National Forest, a large swath of protected land stretching from Yellowstone to Grand Teton, to the southern terminus of the Wind River Range and beyond. Phil was in traumatic cardiac arrest by the time Teton County Search and Rescue delivered him to us in the ambulance. We tried everything we could to save Phil's life—we continued CPR, started IVs, administered epinephrine, inserted a breathing tube, and performed bilateral needle decompressions in case he had two collapsed lungs—but it was futile.

"Blunt force trauma to the head and torso," the coroner would conclude.

Phil was a devoted husband and father of two girls.

The coroner in Jackson was on another assignment, so we had to transport Phil back to the town in the ambulance. There were three of us on the call that afternoon, but only two seats up front in the cab.

"Sorry," my captain said. "You'll have to ride in the back with Phil."

It was a one-hour trip through Grand Teton back to Jackson. My attention kept bouncing between the horrors inside the ambulance and the beauty outside of it. Phil lay on the gurney next to my seat, his snowsuit cut and splayed open to expose his chest and extremities. The air in the ambulance was heavy and smelled of sweat and copper blood. I opened the window, where outside, snow squalls leapt and danced in the crisp, clean air, and bison stood behind the buck-rail fence at Elk Ranch Flats. Deep lacerations covered Phil's head, and the left side of his skull was deformed. He had a small hole in his head from the handlebars. The mountains were covered with clouds. Phil's eyes were wide and his pupils fixed and dilated. As we passed the National Elk Refuge, red horse-drawn sleighs moved over the white snow through herds of brown elk. Phil's left collar bone was broken, his chest wall pale and sunken, and blood dripped from the IV catheters we'd placed in his torso to treat a collapsed lung. And at Flat Creek—just minutes from the hospital—a trumpeter swan, its neck curved like a white question mark, took flight.

The third incident that weighed on me was a phone call from Zach, the law enforcement ranger I'd worked with at Yellowstone. He and I had attended the Fire Academy together.

"He's gone," said Zach.

"Who?" I asked.

"You didn't hear?"

I hadn't. Zach told me that Scott, the lead instructor who'd trained and inspired us all had committed suicide. Memories came flooding back and I could still hear Scott encouraging us before our final live fire scenario in the burn box. "Team 3, are you a go for live fire?"

Each first responder inhabited his or her own haunted house, and these were just a few of my ghosts. I didn't have any thoughts of harming myself or others; I wasn't abusing any substances, and my sleep was improving, so I didn't feel like I needed professional help.

But I was in a dark place after finding Samantha, and then eight days later, my uncle Paul passed away suddenly. Growing up, we used to camp with Paul and his family at Fundy National Park in Canada. The area was home to the highest tides on earth, and we had flocked to the beaches to play hide-and-seek among the "flowerpot" rock formations.

I traveled to Florida for my uncle's funeral, and when I returned to Jackson Hole, everything came to a head. We were training on vehicle extrication, and we had obtained a few cars to practice cutting up, using hydraulic tools. There were three vehicles: an old Toyota Camry, a Honda minivan, and a 2005 Chevy Cobalt.

It can't be, I thought as I approached.

It was. Samantha's family hadn't wanted her car back. The police had no use for it, so why not remove *Desert Solitaire* and her climbing shoes, cover the crimson stain on the driver's seat with a car wash towel, and donate the vehicle to the nearest rescue agency?

"Are you kidding me?" I said as the horrifying memories from the call came flooding back. "That's so messed up!"

I stormed off, and another firefighter, unaware of my history with the vehicle, called after me. "What's wrong?" he yelled. "It's just a car!"

As anger and sadness coursed through me, I knew I needed to own up to my suffering and try to help myself.

SOMETHING FOR THE PAIN

WHEN I BEGAN MY WILD ADVENTURE at Yellowstone, my goal was to become an all-hazards responder so I could serve my country and save lives. And since starting as a paramedic with the National Park Service and working for Jackson Hole Fire/EMS, I'd gotten certified as a structural and wildland firefighter; became proficient in search and rescue; earned hazardous materials operations and awareness credentials; became a fire apparatus driver and operator so I could drive the fire truck and run its highly complex pump; and graduated from a Counter Narcotics and Terrorism Operational Medical Support course so I could insert with a SWAT team during a mass violence incident and do "the greatest good, for the greatest number."

But could I help myself?

The rates of depression for firefighters and police officers were more than five times the civilian average, and suicide killed more first responders in 2018 than line-of-duty deaths. This meant going home for us was more dangerous than coming to work. As I read these studies, I thought about all my friends who'd left the first responder profession. How many cases of burnout were just misdiagnosed PTSD? All I knew for sure was that I was hurting. Like my injured patients on the ambulance who begged for something for the pain, I needed to get help. But I felt ashamed. *Was I alone? Who could I talk to? Was I normal?*

I began my healing by first acknowledging my suffering and owning it. *I've seen some horrific things. I am in pain, and I'm going to do whatever it takes and work hard to get through this*, I thought. Next, I turned to journaling, a practice that had always helped me deal with problems in the past.

I began by writing about the incident with Samantha, the ride in the back of the ambulance with Phil, the sadness I felt about Scott's suicide, and all the other traumatic incidents I'd been a part of. Details of these calls filled my notebook, but over time, the calls lost some of their horror, as isolated and fragmented memories and images formed themselves into sentences, and my own personal narrative emerged. I realized I'd spoken of these calls to coworkers, family, and friends but had never really told the whole story to the most important person: me.

I also pored over articles and listened to podcasts about PTSD and learned a few very important things: I wasn't alone. The price of working as a first responder was grief, and I should expect to experience the full range of emotions. Any feeling was valid. I shouldn't try to normalize these horrific experiences because they were anything but normal, and each trauma was specific to each person, meaning what affected me might not affect someone else and vice versa.

Thanks to these enlightened articles and podcasts, my feelings felt validated and my own posttraumatic stress struggles started to make sense in my mind. But I still felt the trauma in my body: the racing heart, sudden sweating episodes, and intrusive flashbacks. I tried to push out these lingering feelings from my system with long runs and grueling gym workouts. Unsurprisingly, I ended up overdoing it and tweaking my neck, so I decided to take a hot yoga class one Friday morning.

I was in a bad mood as I sat down. The teacher that day was a woman in her late twenties named Faith. She wore her brown hair in a bun, Lululemon everything, and carried a green smoothie in a glass jar.

What does she know about pain? I thought to myself, assuming her definition of tragedy was when Starbucks ran out of chai.

I assumed Faith would have nothing of relevance to teach me, yet as she began class, I soon felt as if she were instructing me alone. The theme of the class was turning pain into gold. "In Japan, there is this practice known as *Kintsugi*, in which broken pottery bowls are repaired with gold lacquer," she told us, reading from her journal. "The flaw is seen as a unique piece of the object's history, which adds to its beauty."

When Faith asked us to select something in our lives that had been causing us pain, I immediately thought of Samantha and her Chevy Cobalt.

"Today we will work with turning that pain into gold," Faith continued. "The writer Ernest Hemingway said, 'The world breaks everyone and afterward many are strong at the broken places.'"

For the next forty-five minutes, I didn't think about Samantha's suicide. Frankly, I was just trying not to pass out. The yoga studio was heated to 105 degrees, and as we performed a flowing series of intense postures and balancing poses, sweat stung my eyes, and my muscles screamed. But as class neared its conclusion and Faith had us assume pigeon pose, a seated hip opener, details from the call with Samantha bubbled up.

Samantha hunched forward in her car.
Her blonde hair covering her face.
The entry wound on her right temple and exit on the left.
The puddle of congealed blood in her lap.
The green flatline on the cardiac monitor.

"We hold our emotions in our hips," Faith explained. "So breathe through whatever arises."

As feelings of grief coursed through me, I wanted to grab my yoga mat and get the hell out of there. But every time I thought of racing for the door, Faith would say something like, "Stay with it and breathe" or quote the Persian poet Rumi, "The cure for the pain is in the pain."

I took the remainder of class one moment at a time, breath by breath, and got through it. I'd heard from one podcast that accessing the inner compartment of our trauma was like opening a shaken soda can: pain shoots out initially in a raging torrent and then dissipates with time.

"Peace does not mean to be in a place where there is no noise, trouble, or hard work," Faith said at the end of class, "it means to be in the midst of those things and still be calm in your heart."

"Thank you," I said to Faith on my way out. "I really needed that."

I felt bad for judging Faith based on her appearance. I was certain from the way she taught that she'd overcome some tough things in her life too. *No matter how perfect someone's life looks*, I thought, *everybody's going through something.*

• • • • • • •

I finally felt like I was healing.

Despite this, when I was dispatched to a call at a concession-aire dorm for an employee who'd attempted suicide by ingesting pills, I was seized with worry. *I can't lose another one*, I thought to myself, as I pulled on a pair of exam gloves and we raced toward the scene with lights and sirens.

We found Beatrice seated at a picnic table outside her dorm. She was a Latina woman in her early twenties, and she was distraught over a fight with her boyfriend. Her black hair was disheveled, and trails of mascara tears ran down her cheeks.

As Jeff and I slowly approached—so as to not overwhelm Beatrice—Wes, Grand Teton's Battalion Chief of Fire/EMS, informed us that she had taken forty cough and cold medication pills and twenty nicotine lozenges.

"Were you trying to hurt yourself?" I asked her.

"Yes," Beatrice whispered.

I was relieved to find her alert and oriented and able to walk with assistance. But the call was still very serious. While the cold medication pills had a relatively low toxicity—and wouldn't cause much harm outside of some nausea and vomiting—the nicotine could cause a dangerous overdose. Following the initial stimulating effects, which raised blood pressure and heart rate, the depressive effects kicked in, plummeting those same vital signs and potentially leading to cardiac arrest. Most importantly, the call was critical because it was a cry for help. In her torment, she'd swallowed whatever pills she could get her hands on. What if she found stronger pills in the future?

We assisted her into the ambulance, and I allowed a friend of hers to sit next to her. A fight with her boyfriend had set Beatrice off, so the last thing she needed was to be in the back of the ambulance with another guy. Ideally, we would've had a female EMT or paramedic seated in the back with her, but none were on duty that day.

As we started rolling toward St. John's Medical Center in Jackson, I gave Beatrice some Zofran for nausea and started an IV, through which I administered a thousand milliliters of saline. "The solution for the pollution is dilution," I recalled from paramedic school. Then, with the medical interventions in place, I focused on the most important treatment, compassion.

I let Beatrice know she wasn't alone and that all her feelings were valid. I told her that I'd learned to read people from working as a firefighter and paramedic. "And I can tell you've got a lot of gifts. You have so much potential and good in you," I said. "You're just going through a difficult time right now."

Some suicidal patients were so altered or far gone that there was no way to reach them. But I sensed a window of opportunity with Beatrice. Today, this low point might be the darkness just before the dawn.

At first, Beatrice barely listened. She just stared blankly out the ambulance window as we zoomed across the sagebrush meadows. But then I could see her taking in the landscape, her eyes darting left to right with the passing trees and then lifting up toward the horizon as we passed the Cathedral Group—Grand Teton, Mount Owen, and Teewinot. And then, suddenly, she blinked twice, as if waking up, and her attention was in the ambulance with us. Since she was listening, I told her again that we were all there for her, that her feelings were valid, and I expressed my belief that she'd get through this, that she had a lot of good in her. I told her everything I wish I could've said to Samantha and my fire instructor Scott and everything I was, in many ways, still telling myself.

Beatrice nodded and said, "Thank you," softly. And then, for the first time that afternoon, I saw something new in her eyes. Hope.

THE CALL OF THE SUMMER

"WHAT HAPPENED?" I asked, cradling an unconscious nine-year-old girl named Eliza at Jackson Lake Lodge.

"Well Eliza had chicken soup last night," her mom began frantically, "and she ate the normal amount, maybe a little less because it was the kind with the thin noodles, and she prefers the thick. Anyways, she woke up feeling a little cold this morning and—"

I cut the hysterical woman off. This wasn't the information I needed first.

"What happened right now? Why is she like this?"

Eliza's dad said she'd had two seizures that morning and had received 7.5 milligrams of the sedative Versed to stop them.

"How much?" I asked incredulously.

Mom explained, "7.5 milligrams, because she weighs seventy-five pounds."

I could barely comprehend the magnitude of this medical math error. The pediatric dose for Versed was 0.1 milligrams per kilogram, up to an adult dose of 2.5 milligrams. Whoever had given Eliza the Versed had not only failed to convert her weight into kilograms but also given her three times the adult dose. "Children are killed by misplaced decimal points," my instructor at paramedic school had taught us.

"Eliza," I said, shaking her shoulders. "Can you open your eyes for me?"

No response.

"Let's get moving," I said to Jeff, picking the girl up in my arms and hurrying to the ambulance.

I ran more calls for pediatric patients during my time with the National Park Service than at any other point in my career: asthma attacks, allergic reactions, campfire burns, bloody noses, insect bites, broken bones, and splinters. One three-year-old swallowed the button battery from his father's watch; a little girl confused her mother's sleeping pills for breath mints; an unrestrained baby boy fell out of his car seat and hit his head on the concrete when his dad opened the door. And there was one instance where a can of bear spray was fired on a school bus packed full of elementary kids returning from a field trip.

Pediatric calls were always a challenge. Kids were notorious for showing vague changes in their mental status and vital signs, only to suddenly deteriorate and become critical. There were also the anatomical differences: a child's head was larger in proportion to the body than an adult, which made them more susceptible to trauma, especially after a fall. A child's smaller size and proportionally lesser amount of blood also put them in greater danger of going into shock or bleeding to death from a wound.

Children had larger tongues and smaller airways with more soft tissue, making them more susceptible to foreign body and airway obstructions. The temperature control mechanism on pediatric patients was also unstable, and they dehydrated easier. As opposed to adults, who show signs of shock with early changes in heart rate and blood pressure, kids compensated much longer before suddenly crashing—and cardiac arrest was usually secondary to respiratory failure.

To combat this, we were taught to form our general impression of the child at the door, basically at arm's length, before approaching. To take a moment to look at the child's ABCs—appearance, breathing, and circulation—from across the room. Did the child appear alert, agitated, sleepy, or unresponsive? Was the child's airway open? How was the child's breathing? What was the child's respiratory rate? What were their skin color and condition? As in many emergency situations, using checklists and reference charts could help.

But that afternoon at Jackson Lake Lodge with Eliza, I didn't need a pediatric vital sign reference chart to know she was near death. It was obvious from her pale, floppy appearance. Was this due to her seizure? Some other neurological condition? Or was it due to the massive medication error? Frankly, at that moment, I didn't care about the cause—I simply had to treat the symptoms. Fast.

Sandy, our college EMT intern, hurried to the ambulance to drive, and Jeff and Brennan hopped in back with me.

"Code 3 to the Moran baseball field," I yelled.

"You got it," Sandy replied, activating the emergency lights and sirens.

After a quick consultation moments earlier, Jeff, Brennan, and I had agreed to call a helicopter. Along with the med error, Eliza had suffered multiple unexplained seizures that morning, and the drive time to the hospital in Jackson Hole was over an hour long.

As we raced toward the Moran district of the park, we inserted a rubber, trumpet-like nasopharyngeal airway into her right nostril to keep her airway open as we continued high-flow oxygen. Eliza felt warm, so we removed her outer layer of clothes on the small chance her seizures were caused by a fever. Next, we took a set of vital signs, checked her blood sugar, and attempted to start an IV, but it wasn't happening. Neither Jeff nor I could place an IV in her tiny, spiderlike veins.

Any port in a storm, I thought, grabbing the intraosseous drill to place a needle in her shin bone for access. I swabbed below her knee with an alcohol prep pad and was just about to drill when Eliza started crying.

"It's OK, Eliza," I said. "We're driving to meet your parents now."

Since we were minutes from the Moran baseball field by then, I set the IO drill down and focused all my energies on comforting the little girl. The flight team was waiting when we arrived. Using our combined efforts, we placed an IV and further stabilized Eliza before her flight to Eastern Idaho Regional Medical Center. There, she'd make a full recovery, but all that Versed certainly didn't help.

• • • • • • •

The real call of the summer didn't arrive by alarm tones or phone but by text message. "Are you available for a search and rescue up on Disappointment Peak? —Miller."

"Miller" was Mike Miller, a Jenny Lake district ranger. He had had command over almost every search-and-rescue mission in the Tetons for the last decade. For months, I'd been pleading to go out on a SAR with a "put me in, coach" persistence, and now my time had come.

I immediately called the Jenny Lake Rescue cache and told Mike I was available, then listened to the specifics of the mission: a twenty-year-old French Canadian from Quebec named Etienne had been hiking alone on Disappointment Peak, a towering 11,617-foot spire, when he fell fifty feet, losing consciousness briefly and breaking bones. Etienne had managed to call 9-1-1, but his phone battery died moments before dispatch could determine his exact location. Fortunately for Etienne, several NPS employees who worked in vegetation (meaning they helped remove noxious weeds and exotic species like thistle and the New Zealand mud snail) were out hiking the peak on their day off and had spotted him. They'd radioed the Jenny Lake search-and-rescue team with Etienne's location. The Jenny Lakers initially wanted to perform a short-haul hoist rescue with the helicopter to save Etienne, but a fierce wind had kicked up, grounding the chopper.

"So we need to do a carryout, and I want you to be the lead advanced life support provider," Mike concluded. "Can you help us?"

I had sprained my ankle badly a few days prior, but I didn't hesitate. "I'm in," I said, grabbing my go bag and racing to my truck.

Thirty minutes later, I pulled up to the Jenny Lake Rescue Cache in Lupine Meadows, where the yellow SAR helicopter sat like a bird with a broken wing, defeated, on the ground. As I hurried inside, the room buzzed with all the activity of a SAR in progress—a coffee pot brewing, radios crackling with recon traffic, and yellow-shirted SAR team members assembling gear.

Mike, the Jenny Lake supervisory ranger, handed me a small, black Pelican case full of narcotics and a kit containing everything I'd need to start an IV. He explained that an off-duty Jenny Lake ranger and his wife were already on-scene with the patient and that he'd sent a team of two ahead of us with the wheeled litter and a basic life support bag.

"Right now, Etienne is alert and oriented and complaining of right shoulder pain and left knee pain," Mike added. "They're attempting to move him down to the trail near Amphitheater Lake."

My team would consist of myself and two others: Josh and Brennan, the Jenny Lake law-enforcement and climbing ranger. Josh worked for the trail crew in Grand Teton during the summer and made snow at the Jackson Hole Mountain Resort in the winter. He was a rugged guy with dark, unruly hair and a wooly beard.

"Nothing like getting paid to hike!" Josh exclaimed as a ranger dropped us off at the trailhead and we started sprinting up. "And save a life!"

"We need to slow down," Brennan said moments later, following closely behind. "We have a *long* day ahead of us."

"I agree," I added, following Brennan. "Gotta pace ourselves!"

The trail to Amphitheater Lake was a strenuous out-and-back 8.9-mile trail with nearly three thousand feet of elevation gain. As we hurried, Brennan warned against flaming out early and reminded us that the hard work really began once we reached the patient. "This is one of the hardest wheeled carryouts in the Tetons. It's 3:00 PM," he said. "We'll be lucky if we're finished by 11:00 tonight!"

"Copy," replied Josh, at the front of the pack. "Slowing down."

"Slowing down," I repeated, though I still needed to *speed up* to stay with him and Brennan.

That's how it went for the next ninety minutes. We kept telling each other to slow down and pace ourselves, yet our legs maintained their fast, frantic pace up the steep trail. We were all aware of the risk of hitting a wall and crashing physically before reaching Etienne, but we also knew we had to move quickly if we could help save his life.

The trail climbed through a mixed conifer forest of pine, spruce, and fir trees for 1.7 miles and then rose steeply through a sparsely wooded mountainside in a series of switchbacks. Far below us, Jackson appeared like a tiny train-set town in the distance. Bradley and Taggart Lakes were two turquoise eyes in sockets of green forest. As I continued up, sweat drenched my shirt, my lungs burned with effort, and my ankle throbbed with pain, but I'd been training for this moment since I was first introduced to search and rescue at Yosemite. This was why I'd logged all those hours trail running up to Columbia Point and Upper Yosemite Falls.

As Brennan, Josh, and I sprinted up the trail, we used conversation to distract us from the searing August heat, hot wind, and steep slope: *Were Instagram and geotagging killing once-secret destinations like the hidden trail to Delta Lake? What were the pros and cons of charging people for search and rescue? And did operators like Navy SEALs really need to be so cocky?*

"Definitely," replied Brennan.

"Yes, but arrogance can lead to tunnel vision and mistakes," offered Josh.

I said that I wanted to work alongside great team members—someone like Stephen Curry who wasn't afraid to take the final buzzer-beater shot, but also someone who wasn't afraid to solicit input and pass the ball if the situation demanded it. "I think someone can be both supremely confident in their abilities and also be humble."

"Confident but not cocky," said Brennan over his shoulder. "I like it!"

While it was late August, you could see hints of fall in the crisp, browning leaves and the abundance of animals, like ruffed grouse, mule deer, and pikas—small rabbit-like creatures with a distinct call—out foraging for food.

"Snake!" Josh suddenly called out, stepping over a slithering black rope on the dirt trail.

I jumped.

"Don't worry," Josh said, continuing on. "Just a nonvenomous wandering garter snake."

After three and a half miles of tough uphill, we rounded a corner and stumbled upon the rescue team. The wheeled litter had met up with another ranger, his wife, and Etienne moments before, and began slowly hiking down.

I quickly got a hand-off report and immediately turned my attention to Etienne. "Je parle un peu français," I began. "Je m'appelle Kevin."

"Ah bien!" he replied with a smile. "Je m'appelle Etienne!"

When Etienne smiled, I knew I could continue my assessment, albeit now in English. *Can you tell me where you are right now? What year is it? What hurts? Do you remember the fall? Did you lose consciousness? Do you have any medical problems? Allergies?*

Based on his answers, I determined that Etienne's airway, breathing, circulation, and mental status were good, so I focused on his injuries. He had discomfort in his right shoulder and left knee and had multiple abrasions on his arms and legs. I had planned on starting an IV and giving him Fentanyl, but surprisingly, Etienne didn't want any narcotics and stated his pain was well-controlled with the ibuprofen the ranger had given him on-scene.

"You sure?" I asked again. "It's a long, bumpy ride down."

"I'm good," Etienne replied.

"Do you feel nauseous at all?" I inquired.

"No, sir."

Etienne's refusal made me realize that sometimes not performing an intervention was the hardest thing for an advanced life support provider. I thought through the logistics, time, and tactics of the call again. I knew that starting an IV right then would destroy the momentum of the call, slow us down, and I'd be working in a dirty, dusty environment. Basic life support was working, and adding advanced life support at this stage would only complicate matters. There were a lot of interventions I wanted to do for Etienne, but on the trail, I had to limit those to what I absolutely needed to do, right then.

"Let's keep to basic life support now and focus on getting him off the trail," I told the group, "and we'll switch tactics if anything changes."

We quickly bandaged Etienne's knee, placed his right arm and shoulder in a sling and swathe wrap, and assisted him onto the vacuum mattress and then into the wheeled litter.

Instead of the larger wheeled litter I'd used at Yosemite, this one was lightweight and designed to be operated by two people, except when the trail was excessively steep or rocky.

"I'll handle medical," I said to Brennan, "and you coordinate the extraction plan."

"Copy," he replied.

Brennan's plan was to hike Etienne down in the wheeled litter in pairs, switching every ten minutes so as not to exhaust ourselves. He assigned us partners, pairing Josh with Brennan, and me with Andrew, a Jenny Lake climbing intern. Andrew and I took the first shift.

"Water bar!" I yelled as we worked the wheeled litter down the trail a few minutes later and approached a dip in the trail and a line of knee-high rocks positioned sixty degrees across the slope. This drainage feature helped direct water off the trail, but it also presented a significant tripping hazard for a wheeled carryout.

"Water bar, lifting one, two, THREE!" Andrew replied as we lifted Etienne and the wheeled litter up and over the procession of rocks and continued down the trail.

I found navigating the wheeled litter down the trail and around, up, and over the rocks terribly hard. I was positioned in the front, steering, and Andrew was in back, occasionally slowing us down with a hand brake. To proceed, we were at once moving down the trail and resisting the heavy, forward momentum of the litter, which threatened to run me over at any moment. And then there were those water bars, which seemed to appear every fifty yards and required us to lift both the litter and the person inside it. Every muscle in my arms and back screamed with effort. It felt as if I were doing triceps dips at the gym in a weight vest with a gorilla on my back.

"The helicopter rescues are the most dramatic," Adam Moore had once said to me, "but wheeled carryouts are often the most work."

As ten minutes of working the litter felt like two hours, I finally understood what he meant.

"Switch!" Brennan hollered as the alarm on his iPhone sounded.

Although my arms and sprained ankle ached with effort and pain that afternoon, I couldn't have been happier to be back on the trails once again. I'd become a paramedic and an all-hazards responder in order to operate in all environments, equally competent in saving lives outdoors and in urban environments. It dawned on me how much I'd grown as a provider—and a person—since that snowy night on the Snowman Trek in the Himalayan Kingdom of Bhutan in 2010, when I'd felt so helpless and unable to assist my client more while she suffered from altitude sickness and dehydration. As I recalled that terrifying night and the prayer I'd made in the looming, 24,035-foot moon shadow of Mount Chomolhari, I felt proud to have kept the promise I'd made with God to dedicate my life to helping people.

Over the past five years, I'd earned a lot of certifications and gained a bunch of experience, but best of all, the journey had led me to an amazing woman named Meaghan, who I met after my last summer in Yellowstone. We were friends for a few years before we fell in love—and would soon get engaged—based upon a mutual interest in travel, adventure, and the outdoors. Like me, Meaghan recognized the importance of community, conservation, and believed that, as Edward Abbey said, "Wilderness is not a luxury, but a necessity of the human spirit."

"Bear!" Brennan suddenly yelled, rousing me from my reverie as he pointed toward a dark shadow just above the trail.

"Hey, bear!" I yelled, alerting him to our presence.

Since arriving in Yellowstone years earlier, I'd had numerous encounters with bruins and now felt comfortable enough to handle an encounter that was safe for both me and the bear.

"Don't worry, it's just a black bear," I said over my shoulder to Etienne, "not a grizzly!"

The bear paid us little regard. The huckleberries were blooming, and the bear looked as if he were in a food coma as our SAR procession raced past.

As we continued down the trail, navigating over rocks and steep sections, I kept Etienne talking in order to continually assess his mental status. Etienne told me he was hitchhiking to national parks across the country, reminding me of another "Dharma Bum," the Beatnik writer and French Canadian Jack Kérouac.

When we passed over a small, wooden bridge, we radioed to the SAR Cache that we were inbound, and twenty minutes later, we met the ambulance at the trailhead.

"Want me to take over the patient?" Adam Moore asked, hopping out of the driver's seat.

The normal procedure was for the SAR team to hand off the patient to the crew on the ambulance. I was exhausted and wanted nothing more than to clean up and crack a beer to celebrate a successful rescue, but I was determined to finish the mission.

"I'll maintain patient care," I replied and then turned to Etienne. "I'm coming to the hospital with you."

As we moved Etienne from the wheeled litter into the ambulance, my work area switched from an austere, trailside environment to a spacious, clean ER on four wheels. Hours ago near Amphitheater Lake, I had to operate on the basis of time, tactics, and the least invasive treatment to prioritize getting Etienne off the trail, whereas now I could work in broader EMS brushstrokes.

"What do you need?" Adam asked, hopping in the patient compartment with me.

"Let's get an updated set of vital signs. Place an IV. Give a fluid bolus, reassess his pain level, and hook him up to the EKG," I replied.

With that, Adam and I jumped into action, and minutes later we were en route to the hospital, twenty minutes away. "St. John's ER," I said and radioed in my patient care report: "Medic 1 with a trauma yellow patient based on the mechanism of a fifty-foot fall."

Once I finished, I quickly turned my attention back to Etienne. I wanted to make sure no afterdrop phenomenon occurred and that he didn't have any new or increased pain, now that the adrenaline from the rescue was wearing off.

At the hospital, Etienne was diagnosed with a shoulder fracture and an open knee fracture that needed immediate surgery, but the doctors were certain he'd make a full recovery and could continue his vagabonding ways once again.

"They'll take good care of you here," I said, shaking Etienne's hand. "Feel better."

"Merci," he replied. "Vous êtes un héros!"

· · · · · · ·

Later, as Adam and I drove back to Grand Teton National Park, we passed the accident scene of the terrible crash just north of Jackson Hole Airport that had claimed three lives a month prior. As I thought about holding my patient Nora's hand—and she mine—just before she died, my eyes welled with tears, and I quickly put on my sunglasses.

"It was a horrific scene," Adam replied when I asked his thoughts about the call where two vehicles hit head-on at fifty-five miles per hour. "But also, our finest hour." Despite the fatalities, Adam spoke about how we'd saved a family that afternoon and the extraordinary interagency response of Grand Teton National Park, Jackson Hole Fire/EMS, law enforcement, and the flight teams on the three helicopters that had transported the surviving patients from Jackson Hole to Eastern Idaho Regional Medical Center.

"There was no *us* and *them* that day," Adam explained, referring to the multiagency response. "There was only *we*."

"There is only we," I repeated softly.

I didn't yet know the exact meaning of what he'd said, but the music resonated.

As we pulled into the park headquarters at the Moose Entrance Station to restock for the next call, I realized picking the call of the summer meant identifying an event in the past, but what my experience with the NPS had given me was a wonderful faith in the future.

The following week, I gave a presentation on EMS within the Park Service to thirty high school students participating in the Youth Conservation Program. They were spending ten weeks learning about the NPS mission and working in the park constructing trails, fixing fences and bridges, and restoring historic structures. Following a lecture on hands-only CPR and bleeding control, I gave them a tour of the apparatus bay, and when I threw open the back doors of the ambulance, their eyes lit up as if seeing Narnia for the first time.

"How do I become a paramedic?" asked a boy from New York.

"I'm hoping to work as a wildlife biologist," added a girl from Wyoming.

"I'll be attending a structure fire academy later this year," a boy from Washington State said proudly.

Other students wanted to work as marine biologists, geologists, doctors, and environmental engineers.

"If you can dream it, you can do it!" I replied, quoting Walt Disney.

Despite the current challenges, I knew the mission of service and stewardship of the National Park Service would continue into the next century and beyond, because the agency would always be full of passionate people like those kids, who were as resilient and rugged as the land we were called upon to protect.

When I got off shift that evening, I changed into my workout gear, tightened the straps on my trail running pack, and jogged up the undulating trail toward Taggart Lake. As I ran, I felt connected to something beautiful and timeless, beyond all comprehension, and much bigger than myself. Purple and red wildflowers danced in the mountain wind. A moose wandered up among the huckleberries on a glacial moraine, and, underfoot, every pebble sat perfectly in its place.

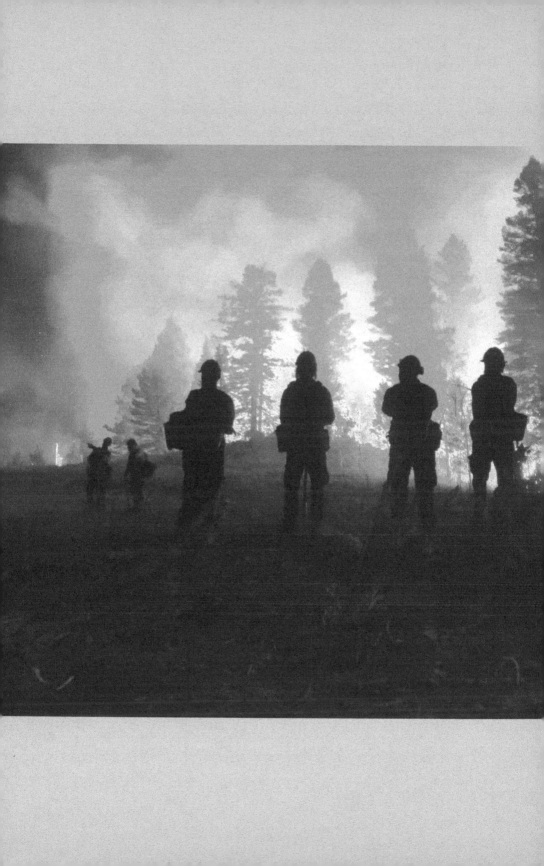

EPILOGUE

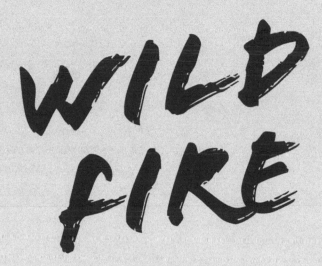

WILD FIRE

Nature is not a place to visit. It is home.

—Gary Snyder

EPILOGUE

WILDFIRE

AS I SAW THE FLAMES cresting over the ridge, I realized with horror that we were about to get overrun by the wildfire for the second time on that hot, chaotic afternoon.

"Get back to the engine," I yelled into my radio, hoping to get the attention of the three firefighters combating the blaze. "We need to evacuate now!"

It was the first big wildland fire I'd responded to since earning my "red card," which allowed me to deploy when a forest was ablaze. That afternoon, I was on shift with Jackson Hole Fire/ EMS and assigned to operate Engine 11. As engineer, my job was to safely drive the truck to the scene and then operate the pump panel, ensuring the firefighters at the nozzle received the water they needed. The pump panel on Engine 11 was located immediately behind the cab, which meant I had a good, elevated spot to watch fire conditions, and that was precisely why I realized we needed to get the hell out of there right that instant.

"Pull back," I hollered again into the radio, which was set to tactical channel 3, so only our crew in the immediate vicinity could hear. "We're going to get burnt over."

I knew this with absolute certainty, because it had nearly happened an hour earlier at the top of the butte, and it was all due to some child's birthday balloons. They must've looked so benign floating in the summer sky, released by some tiny, innocent hand. But then they got tangled in a set of power lines, and the sparks ignited the dry grasses below.

At Station 1 of Jackson Hole Fire/EMS, which sat adjacent to the rodeo grounds, we'd just finished two grueling hours of structure-fire training and were sitting down to lunch when the alarm tones sounded: *The following units respond to a wildland fire: Engine 11, Tender 17, Tender 77, Brush 18, Brush 78, and Duty Officer. This will be a wildfire in the sagebrush, across the street from the Virginian Lodge. . . .*

Captain Joel Conner, firefighters Steve and Manuel, and I threw on our yellow wildland fire brush shirts and green Nomex pants, grabbed our helmets, and quickly responded. Once we arrived at the base of Saddle Butte, we immediately began attacking the blaze with multiple hoselines and the deck gun. This high-flow nozzle sat atop the engine and lobbed five hundred gallons of water per minute towards the fire like a long touchdown pass. But before the torrent reached the blaze, it was intercepted by the fierce wind that blew it sideways and knocked it down. The high temperature, gusting wind, dry vegetation, and low relative humidity had created the perfect storm for a deadly wildland fire, and, though additional units and firefighters continued to arrive, we couldn't catch the blaze.

As the flames tore uphill, we were reassigned to drive to the top of the butte and protect a subdivision of homes. We needed to move so fast that we unscrewed our hoselines and abandoned them on the ground, a technique known as "cutting and running."

By then, the flames were spreading in all directions and threatening homes and businesses near town. Broadway, the main street through Jackson, was closed, and an eerie orange glow hung in the sky. Ashes danced in the air like gray snowflakes.

The road to the top of Saddle Butte was steep and winding and required me to make three- and four-point turns in Engine 11 to navigate around the tight corners, delaying our response. By the time we reached the top of the saddle and positioned ourselves in the dirt lot of a new home being built, turbulent gray smoke was sweeping over the ridge, suggesting the fire was right behind.

Steve and Manuel pulled two hoselines from Engine 11 as Captain Conner shouted for water. From the driver's seat, I quickly engaged the pump, dashed to the panel to charge the hoselines with water, and then leapt from the engine to help. Our goal was to put out the blaze or, at the very least, dampen the vegetation surrounding the home so it wouldn't ignite. However, unbeknownst to all of us, the fire had grown considerably since we'd last laid eyes on it and winds had picked up. We expected to see smoldering flames creeping over the hillside, which we could easily extinguish. But, instead, we were met with a wide, fast-moving flaming front, barreling towards our position like a tidal wave, pummeling us with intense heat, smoke, and ash. Fortunately, the dirt lot saved us all from being burnt by flames, though the air scorched our lungs.

"I can't breathe," yelled Steve, dropping the nozzle and retreating.

"Pull back," I hollered, following him.

Gasping for air and temporarily blinded by the smoke and ash, we stumbled around punch-drunk and short of breath, unable to decide whether we should flee, deploy our aluminum fire shelters, or seek a safe haven in the half-built home immediately behind us.

Suddenly, one of our battalion chiefs roared up in his department-issued Suburban and threw open the side doors. We sprinted over and dove in, crawling over one another to get out of the heat. By then, it was too smoky to drive, so we hunkered down as hot, gusting winds shook the truck.

Thanks to the fast wind and low sagebrush, the wildfire swept past us as quickly as it arrived, leaving an apocalyptic scene of smoldering flames and charred earth.

Inside the battalion chief's rig, we took stock of one another.

"You alright, Steve?" I asked with bloodshot, tearing eyes.

"I'm good," Steve replied, coughing. "How about you, Manuel?"

"Still here," Manuel managed, his nose running with sooty snot.

As we stepped out of the Suburban, I expected to find Engine 11 reduced to a burnt skeleton of its former self, but, surprisingly, it was intact and still operational.

"You guys ready for another assignment?" asked Captain Conner, hurrying up to us.

Given our close call, I expected Steve and Manuel to protest, but they immediately agreed.

"Put us back in," said Steve.

"Payback time," added Manuel.

I couldn't help but be inspired by their courage.

We refilled Engine 11 at a lone hydrant atop the butte—a red beacon of hope in a black, ashy wasteland—then doused a few spot fires before being tasked to protect a sprawling house on the side of the butte. We parked nose-out in a thin driveway, pulled our hoselines, and began dampening down the vegetation surrounding the home to thwart the flames. That's when I saw the smoke and flames fast approaching. I knew if we got overrun this time, it'd be much worse. There was no dirt lot to protect us; we were surrounded by trees—a greater fuel load than the sagebrush—and the fire could easily jump the road, cutting off our exit.

"Fall back!" I screamed again into the radio a third time. "Get to the engine."

Captain Conner, Steve, and Manuel were so busy fighting the blaze that they didn't copy my radio traffic. There was no doubt that they were about to get severely burnt, so I did the one thing assured to get their attention—I cut off their water supply for a split second. As their nozzles suddenly went dry, they immediately looked back at the engine, and I frantically waved them over. Suddenly, they realized the extent of the danger and came sprinting.

"Cut and run," shouted Captain Conner. "Let's get out of here!"

When Captain Conner, Steve, and Manuel hopped in, I hit the gas and tore out as smoke and flames scoured the area.

As we descended down the winding road, Engine 11's three- and four-point turns felt a lot l-o-n-g-e-r and s-l-o-w-e-r, and I kept worriedly looking in my rearview mirror, expecting to see flames.

We eventually made it safely to our assigned staging area halfway down the butte. It was another dirt construction site, larger than the previous, but also surrounded by sagebrush and an abandoned dump truck with two hulking gas tanks. "If those things catch fire next to us, we're toast," I declared. By then, Engine 11 resembled the *Pequod*, the battered whaling ship from *Moby-Dick*. Since we'd "cut and run" multiple times, we were low on hose, and Engine 11's water tank was half empty, drinking water and food were in short supply, and we were all beat and exhausted. Just then, we spotted the fire rounding the butte in the distance and heading toward us once again.

"We need to go," I said, gazing at the smoke and flames.

"The road is closed," replied Manuel.

"But we can't stay here," countered Steve. "We're surrounded by sagebrush and gas tanks."

We found ourselves in a classic "damned if you do, damned if you don't" scenario.

Captain Conner radioed command about our situation and got approval to evacuate down the closed road if we felt comfortable doing so. "But I can't guarantee we won't get caught by flames," Captain Conner added. "And if we do, there's no place for Engine 11 to turn around."

"We can't stay here," Steve said again. "We have to go."

Captain Conner looked at me. "Thoughts?"

"Let's go for it," I said. "Run this gauntlet."

Manuel agreed and we all piled back in. We would handle this obstacle like all the others we'd faced that day: as brothers in a tight-knit crew.

"Don't let me down, ol' boy," I said to Engine 11 as I gunned it.

When we left the construction site, the road followed a series of undulating ridges. We lost sight of the fire, but I could tell by the massive smoke cloud billowing up that it was somewhere just behind the last towering bluff, waiting for us. As we approached our final obstacle, I knew we would either make it or be stuck in the middle of a massive, raging wildfire. My knuckles tightened and whitened on the steering wheel.

"Here we go," I said, speeding up.

"Let's do this," yelled Steve, tightening his seatbelt.

As we rounded the berm, I readied myself to race through an inferno, but suddenly I saw the flames fifty yards above and moving away from us. An aerial assault team of multiple airplanes and helicopters dropping thousands of gallons of water from large buckets had steered the fire away from the road, ensuring us a clear passage.

"We're safe," I hollered as an airplane soared above the butte, releasing a victorious stream of orange flame retardant.

Captain Conner, Steve, and Manuel cheered wildly.

Thanks to the efforts of over a hundred firefighters, two hot shot crews, and the aerial assault team, no one was injured on the fire, and not a single home was lost. At the bottom of Saddle Butte, as I turned on South Milward Street, townspeople and tourists lined the road, cheering and clapping. Seeing them, I felt so honored to work as a first responder and thankful for my journey with the National Park Service and Jackson Hole Fire/EMS.

In that time, I'd learned a lot about becoming an all-hazards responder but also discovered something about our national identity. As I pulled Engine 11 into our incident command post, a large parking lot off Cache Street, there were dozens of fire trucks and personnel from Jackson Hole Fire/EMS, Grand Teton National Park, Teton Village Fire Department, and the US Forest Service and law-enforcement officers from Jackson Hole Police Department and Teton County Sheriff, along with Teton County Emergency Management and Public Works employees—who'd helped direct traffic and placed barricades around town to block access—and a smattering of volunteers cooking lunch to keep everyone well fed and hydrated.

The saying is true, I realized, *There is only we.*

The scene seemed like the perfect summation of working as an all-hazards responder, and all my thoughts of public safety agencies being separated by jurisdiction, mission statement, and service disappeared. We were all part of a single department, serving one great nation.

"God bless, America," I thought and then walked to the food-and-water rehab station to get ready for the next call.

ACKNOWLEDGMENTS

THIS BOOK WOULD NOT HAVE BEEN POSSIBLE without the help of many kind, generous, and creative souls who encouraged me at every stage of the writing and publishing process.

A huge thank you goes to my literary agent, Jane Dystel, and her business partner, Miriam Goderich, who offered invaluable expertise and support at each and every stage of this book's journey. I am so fortunate to work with the best literary agent team in the business.

I am honored that this memoir found a home at Chicago Review Press and feel grateful to be included among its impressive bookshelf of titles and authors. For his enthusiasm and belief in this project, I thank my wonderful, insightful editor, Jerome Pohlen. Thanks also goes to Chicago Review Press's publisher, Cynthia Sherry; Managing Editor Michelle Williams; and Ben Krapohl, for serving as Assistant Project Editor, along with Jon

Hahn for his design work and Stefani Szenda and Sam Ofman for their assistance with marketing and publicity.

I also owe particular recognition to Shannon Jamieson Vazquez, Joeth Zucco, and Brian Wheeler, who read early drafts of the manuscript and offered invaluable feedback, and Karolina Zapal, for her expert copyediting work. Thanks also goes to Dan Long, Jennifer McGrath, Kyle Reyolds, and Bridget and Olivier Teissier, who helped fact-check certain sections and to Bradly J. Boner and Mike Kirby for allowing use of their stunning wildland fire photos.

In the chapter titled "Something for the Pain," the podcast I reference, which has been particularly helpful in my understanding first responder mental health and human performance, is called *PJ Medcast*, hosted by Lt. Col. Stephen Rush, MD. I found Episodes 34, 40–41, 45, 53, 106–107, and 130–132 particularly informative and highly recommend *PJ Medcast* for every first responder. If you're thinking about suicide or are worried about a friend or loved one—or just need emotional support—the Lifeline network is available twenty-four seven, across the United States, at 1-800-273-8255.

I would also like to thank the National Park Service for giving me access to my patient care reports—which had all of the protected personal information (PPI) redacted—to assist in writing this book and the National Parks Conservation Association, which allowed me to reprint parts of an article I wrote for their magazine.

For their inspired and engaged medical direction, mentorship, and passion for emergency medicine, I wish to thank the Medical Directors I've had the pleasure of serving under in the National Park Service: Dr. Luanne Freer, Dr. Ralph Groves, Dr. A.J. Wheeler, and Dr. Will Smith.

ACKNOWLEDGMENTS

Thank you to all the park rangers and volunteers I've had the pleasure, privilege, and honor of working with at Yosemite, Yellowstone, and Grand Teton who work hard every day to keep visitors safe and our national treasures "unimpaired for future generations." Thanks also goes to my fellow firefighters at Jackson Hole Fire/EMS who inspire me daily with their commitment to serve and to other agencies within our local, first responder community: Teton County Search and Rescue, Teton County Sheriff, Jackson Hole Police, and Wyoming Highway Patrol.

Most importantly, my immense gratitude goes to Meaghan for her unbounded support—and for getting me outside to hike, mountain bike, and white-water raft when I needed a break from writing—along with my dear family. Thank you, Mom; Dad; Kristine and Ola Johansson; Sean and Corie Grange; my niece, Lauren; and my nephews Bjorn, Finn, Hunter, and Taylor. I love you all!